SIMPLE PRINCIPLES™
TO EAT SMART AND
LOSE WEIGHT

Alex A. Lluch
Author of Over 3 Million Books Sold!*

Sarah Jang
Weight Loss and Fitness Coach

WS Publishing Group
San Diego, California

Simple Principles™
to Eat Smart and Lose Weight

By Alex A. Lluch and Sarah Jang

Published by WS Publishing Group
San Diego, California 92119
Copyright © 2008 by WS Publishing Group

Designed by WS Publishing Group:
David Defenbaugh

For Inquiries:
Logon to www.WSPublishingGroup.com
E-mail info@WSPublishingGroup.com

ISBN 13: 978-1-934386-10-1

Printed in China

TABLE OF CONTENTS

Introduction

Studies, surveys, and polls consistently show that if Americans could change one thing about themselves, the majority of people would choose to lose weight. What is it about a thin, slender body that captivates so many of us? In addition to the fact that American culture has always put a premium on being thin, those who are at a low or normal weight are much healthier than those who are overweight or obese. Indeed, high cholesterol, high blood pressure, diabetes, stroke, heart disease, and even death are all consequences of being overweight.

Losing weight has major benefits that can improve your way of life. Weight loss can lower the risk of the diseases mentioned above, help you become more active, and also make you look better and feel better about yourself. Although many of us want to be thinner, it is difficult in today's society to make the right choices regarding our health and diet. Food portions in restaurants are larger than ever before, which encourages us to eat more. In addition, our jobs promote sedentary lifestyles;

and fast food, while often unhealthy, is convenient and inexpensive. Many food companies use larger sized portions as a selling point, making the claim that bigger is better. It then becomes the consumer's responsibility to monitor how much he or she eats and to know how much is personally enough. That is where this book comes in: it educates you on weight loss and weight management methods that actually work. It provides 200 simple principles for practicing dietary health, and it arms you with tools to make your weight loss experience easier, more enjoyable, and more likely to succeed.

What is this book about?

This is a book about losing weight. In more depth, it is a book about setting realistic weight loss goals, creating a weight loss plan, staying motivated, learning to plan ahead, and learning ways to maximize your metabolism. It is about figuring out how to curb your appetite, learn portion control skills, explore healthy alternatives to foods you like, and how to stick to your diet when you dine out. It offers information on foods that help you lose weight and how to change your lifestyle to maintain your weight loss. Finally, it contains everything you need to know about maximizing your health, habits, and environment to result in a thinner you.

Who should read this book?

This book is for anyone who wants to successfully lose weight. It is for people who are trying to lose weight for the first time. This book will give you tools, habits, and ideas to start your weight loss journey off on the right foot. It is also for people who have tried unsuccessfully in the past to lose weight. There are certainly many people out there who have failed in their quest for losing weight. According to the National Institutes of Health, a whopping 98 percent of people who lose weight gain it back within five years. Perhaps even more astonishing, 90 percent gain back even more weight than they lost.

There are three main reasons why people fail to lose weight and keep it off. First, people may have unreasonable goals. Dieters can become discouraged when they fail to meet unrealistic expectations. Second, people may quit dieting when they find extreme weight loss programs too difficult to maintain. Third, they may not understand that sustained weight loss occurs when simple changes are consistently applied to their daily life. This book provides 200 hints, tips, and ideas that will allow you to address these issues and finally realize your weight loss goals.

This book is for people who want to:
- Lose any amount of weight
- Create a weight loss plan
- Learn to stick to their diet during special occasions
- Curb their cravings
- Learn portion control skills
- Learn healthy ways to cook their favorite dishes
- Increase their metabolism
- Create an environment that is conducive to weight loss
- Adopt the habits of slim people
- Learn what colors and sounds facilitate weight loss
- Learn to love working out
- Set goals and chart their weight loss success
- Boost their self-esteem
- Lose those final, stubborn 5 pounds

- Think and act like a thin person
- Stay motivated during weight-loss plateaus and setbacks

Last, this book is for people who want to flip to a page that applies to their situation and find a quick inspirational and informational tip.

Why should you read this book?

Well, you were drawn to the title, so you should read this book! Even if you think you already know how to lose weight, there is something in here for you. In truth, no one can get enough help when they attempt to diet. Even if you already know that eating better and exercising will help you lose weight, this book contains numerous tips, hints, ideas, and statistics that will help you reach your goal weight faster and more enjoyably than if you were to do so on your own. You should read this book because it combines old wisdom with new ideas into easy-to-read simple principles. Here are some questions to ask yourself if you are wondering whether this book will help you reach your weight-loss goals:

- Are you tired of unsuccessful weight loss attempts?
- Have you ever lost weight and then gained it back?
- Do you have trouble staying motivated when dieting?
- Do you find it difficult to exercise?
- Do you have trouble sticking to your diet in restaurants?
- Do you feel you do not have enough time to exercise?
- Is it impossible for you to control your cravings?
- Do you tend to eat healthy foods but in large amounts?
- Would you like to learn how modifying your environment can help you lose weight?
- Have you ever wanted to boost your metabolism?
- Do you want to learn which foods help you lose weight?
- Have you ever wondered why some people can lose weight easily, without even trying?

These are just a few of the 200 topics covered in this book. If any of these questions resonate with you, then you should read this book. The principles contained in this book are thoroughly supported with statistical information from researched studies. Its size makes it easy to keep with you for easy reference in the middle of the day or for a thorough read when you have more time.

THE ETERNAL STRUGGLE TO LOSE WEIGHT

More than half of American adults today are overweight, with one-third considered obese. America's weight problem has become a serious issue because of the increasing number of diseases linked to being overweight, such as high cholesterol, high blood pressure, diabetes, stroke, and heart disease. Such diseases can reduce your quality of life and, in some cases, lead to death. In America, obesity causes roughly 300,000 deaths each year. Furthermore, the health care costs of adults who are obese continue to rise, making being overweight an expensive problem in addition to an unhealthy one. Several factors can contribute to being overweight, including family genetics, the growing portion sizes of food, and the tendency to overeat. The most common way to determine whether or not a person is obese is to determine their Body Mass Index, or BMI. This is a ratio of a person's height and weight. When a person's BMI is over 25, he or she can be considered overweight (see page 15 to learn how to calculate your BMI). Unfortunately,

BMIs over 25 are an increasing trend in America's health statistics. We are a nation whose waistline is expanding and will continue to grow unless we take control of our eating and exercise habits.

Why is it so difficult to lose weight?

As most people know, losing weight is an incredibly difficult endeavor. But why is that? There are a few simple reasons. First and foremost, food is delicious! Eating is one of the most pleasurable activities known to man. In reality, many of us eat, and choose what we eat, based on the fact that we like to do so. The way foods taste and smell, the texture they have in our mouths, the large variety of delicious food and high-calorie drinks available, coupled with the sociable activity we engage in when we sit down for a meal with others, all make it very difficult to control what we eat.

A second reason it is difficult to lose weight stems from our love of food. Our appetite causes us to eat when we are not hungry; to overeat because we like how food tastes; to crave foods that are bad for us; and to substitute eating for other activities when we are bored or restless. Our love of eating causes us to forget the primary biological reasons we are supposed to eat. This makes it difficult to control ourselves when presented with the foods we most love.

A final reason why it is difficult to lose weight is because of the way many modern foods are prepared. Indeed, many foods come processed, packaged, and with higher amounts of sodium, fat, carbohydrates, and calories than ever before. But the main obstacle for American dieters remains fast food. According to a 2005 CBS study titled *How and Where America Eats*, 45 percent of Americans eat fast food for dinner at least 1 night a week. Americans have always had a love affair with fast food because of its convenience and low price. But fast food repeatedly proves to be bad for your waistline, sometimes containing as much as twice the amount of calories and fat a homemade sandwich, salad, or burger would have.

And even when diners chose regular restaurants over fast food, they still consume more calories than if they cooked a meal themselves. Of course, restaurant food is cooked primarily with your palate in mind, not your waistline. Chefs go to great lengths to include sauces, batters, and other calorie-laden accessories to dishes to improve their flavor and presentation. As a result, restaurant dishes have more calories, fat, and sodium than do dishes prepared at home and also tend to be served in larger portions. CBS found that 27 percent of Americans eat in a restaurant at least one night a week, another reason for our nation's expanding waistline.

What do you need to lose weight successfully?

The most important reasons to start a weight-loss program are to look and feel great and to reduce the risk of health complications, such as heart disease and diabetes. Before you start, however, it is important to assess your current health status. It is just as important to define your current starting point as it is to set your final goal. To determine your starting point, you must assess how much you weigh now and how much weight you need to lose. There are three things you need in order to determine your overall physical condition: your height and weight measurements, waist size, and Body

Mass Index (BMI). A final piece of information that you need to determine your weight-loss goals is your family history.

Your Body Mass Index (BMI) is a measure of body fat based on height and weight that applies to all adult men and women. It allows people to assess their current physical status using a standard to compare it to. We need a standard because body composition can vary greatly from individual to individual. Two people who possess the same height and weight can have different bone structure and varying percentages of muscle and fat. Therefore, your weight alone is not the only factor in assessing your risk for weight-related health issues. Your BMI also can help indicate whether or not your health is at risk.

For adults 18 years and older, the first step is to measure your height and weight. Then, plug those two numbers into the following formula to find your BMI.

$$BMI = \left(\frac{\text{Weight in Pounds}}{(\text{Height in inches}) \times (\text{Height in inches})} \right) \times 703$$

That is, a person who weighs 160 lbs. and is 5'8" tall has a BMI of 24.3.

$$BMI = \left(\frac{160}{68 \times 68} \right) \times 703 = 24.3$$

Body Mass Index Chart

BMI	19	20	21	22	23	24	25	26	27	28	29	30	31	32	33	34	35
Height								weight in pounds									
4'10"	91	96	100	105	110	115	119	124	129	134	138	143	148	153	158	162	167
4'11"	94	99	104	109	114	119	124	128	133	138	143	148	153	158	163	168	173
5'	97	102	107	112	118	123	128	133	138	143	148	153	158	163	158	174	179
5'1"	100	106	111	116	122	127	132	137	143	148	153	158	164	169	174	180	185
5'2"	104	109	115	120	126	131	136	142	147	153	158	164	169	175	180	186	191
5'3"	107	113	118	124	130	135	141	146	152	158	163	169	175	180	186	191	197
5'4"	110	116	122	128	134	140	145	151	157	163	169	174	180	186	192	197	204
5'5"	114	120	126	132	138	144	150	156	162	168	174	180	186	192	198	204	210
5'6"	118	124	130	136	142	148	155	161	167	173	179	186	192	198	204	210	216
5'7"	121	127	134	140	146	153	159	166	172	178	185	191	198	204	211	217	223
5'8"	125	131	138	144	151	158	164	171	177	184	190	197	203	210	216	223	230
5'9"	128	135	142	149	155	162	169	176	182	189	196	203	209	216	223	230	236
5'10"	132	139	146	153	160	167	174	181	188	195	202	209	216	222	229	236	243
5'11"	136	143	150	157	165	172	179	186	193	200	208	215	222	229	236	243	250
6'	140	147	154	162	169	177	184	191	199	206	213	221	228	235	242	250	258
6'1"	144	151	159	166	174	182	189	197	204	212	219	227	235	242	250	257	265
6'2"	148	155	163	171	179	186	194	202	210	218	225	233	241	249	256	264	272
6'3"	152	160	168	176	184	192	200	208	216	224	232	240	248	256	264	272	279

Healthy	Overweight	Obese

You can also use the chart on the left to calculate your BMI. Locate your height in the left column and then move across the row to your weight. The number in the top row is your BMI.

If your BMI falls within the range of 19 to 24.9, you are considered healthy. If your BMI is less than 18.5, you are considered underweight. If your BMI lands from 25 to 29.9, you are considered overweight and have an increased risk of developing health problems. Finally, if your BMI is 30 or above, you are considered obese. If you fall into the last two categories, it is essential to start or manage your weight loss program.

The second factor in evaluating your weight is your waist size. Use a tape measure to calculate your waist circumference below your rib cage and above your belly button. Your waist measurement determines whether or not you have the tendency to carry fat around your midsection. A higher waist size may indicate a greater risk for weight-related health issues such as high blood pressure, type 2 diabetes, and coronary artery disease. You have an increased health risk for developing serious chronic illness if your waist size is more than 35 inches for women and 40 inches for men.

Risk of Associated Disease According to BMI and Waist Size

Body Mass Index		Waist less than or equal to 40" Men 35" Women	Waist greater than 40" Men 35" Women
18 or less	Underweight	N/A	N/A
19-24	Normal	N/A	N/A
25-29	Overweight	Increased	High
30-35	Obese	High	Very High
over 35	Obese	Very High	Very High

If your weight indicates that you are at a higher risk for health problems, consult your primary care physician to determine safe and effective ways to improve your health. Even moderate amounts of weight loss, around five to ten percent of your weight, can have long lasting health benefits if you can keep the pounds off.

A third factor in determining your current health status is knowing your personal history and family background. In addition to shedding light on possible health risks, your family history can tell you if you are likely to have a particularly low or high metabolism, which will affect the ease with which you are able to lose weight. Knowing your family history will also allow you to choose a diet that accommodates any dietary needs you may have. Make sure you choose a weight-loss program that matches your personal dietary needs, including diabetes, allergies, high blood pressure, high cholesterol, high blood sugar, heart problems, or respiratory illness. A history of family illness doesn't mean that you can't lose weight, but you do want to make sure you account for such factors as you plan your weight-loss program.

Finally, before beginning your weight-loss journey, you should also investigate behaviors that may have led to your current weight situation, such as emotional triggers, guilt-based eating, and stress snacking. Changing these habits requires adjusting your attitude toward food. Begin by understanding the situations and emotional triggers that lead to overeating.

Let's take a look at some common behaviors:

Are you compelled to eat as an emotional response to your thoughts and feelings? If you eat when you're upset, frustrated, angry, lonely, or tired, the answer most likely is yes. Food feels like the perfect temporary solution, that is, until it is finished, and then guilt sets in because the food choice may not have been healthy. Try to choose other behaviors as an emotional response, such as taking a walk or calling a friend.

Do you eat when you are not hungry because you think you should? Sometimes the time of day is enough encouragement to eat a meal or a quick snack, despite a lack of actual physical hunger. Instead, learn to listen to your body. You should resist the urge to eat when you are not truly hungry.

Do you feel guilty leaving food on your plate? Perhaps when you were a child, you were told to finish all of the food on your plate. This sense of guilt should no longer gauge how much food you should eat. It is acceptable to stop eating when you feel full.

Do you make poor food choices because of peer pressure? It is far easier to go with the flow when those around you are eating unhealthy foods. It takes self-control and determination to follow your weight loss plan at social gatherings or all-you-can-eat buffets. Congratulate yourself when you stick to your plan and successfully fend off unhealthy snack urges.

Do you eat out of boredom? Food can become a time-filler when you are bored. Don't fall into this trap! Try to motivate yourself and choose a fun and interesting activity as an alternative to snacking. If you are otherwise occupied with an activity where food is not involved, it will be easier to wait for your regularly scheduled meal.

Calculating Your Daily Calorie Allowance

Any diet plan should require you to calculate your daily calorie allowance. The following equation will help you figure out your basal metabolic rate, or BMR, the extra calories you expend based on your activity level, and the number of calories you need to deduct to lose weight. To calculate your daily calorie allowance, the BMR formula below uses the variables of height, weight, age, and gender.

Step 1: Use the following equation to calculate your BMR: (Please note that this formula only applies to adults.)

Women BMR = 655 + (4.3 x weight in pounds) + (4.7 x height in inches) - (4.7 x age in years)

Men BMR = 66 + (6.3 x weight in pounds) + (12.9 x height in inches) - (6.8 x age in years)

Step 2: Select one of the following equations to factor in your activity level. To determine your total daily calorie needs, choose the appropriate activity level and multiply your BMR accordingly:

Sedentary (little or no exercise):
Calorie-Calculation = BMR x 1.2

Lightly active (light exercise/activity 1-3 days/week):
Calorie-Calculation = BMR x 1.375

Moderately active (moderate exercise/activity 3-5 days/week):
Calorie-Calculation = BMR x 1.55

Very active (hard exercise/activity 6-7 days a week):
Calorie-Calculation = BMR x 1.725

Extra active (very hard exercise/activity, physical job or sports conditioning):
Calorie-Calculation = BMR x 1.9

For example, if your BMR is 1,500 and you are sedentary, you would multiply your BMR (1,500) by 1.2 = 1,800.

The result of this calculation is the number of calories you can eat every day and maintain your current weight.

Step 3: To lose weight, you need to create a calorie deficit by reducing your calories below your maintenance level. Or you can keep your calories the same and increase your activity above your current level. If you want to lose a pound a week, you need to subtract 500 calories from your daily allowance through either diet, exercise, or both.

Maximizing the Benefits
of This Book

Always keep this book handy. Put it in the glove box of your car. Stick it in the top drawer of your desk at work. Lay it on your nightstand before bed. Keep it in your briefcase or purse when you visit restaurants. Keep it in your gym bag. This book is written to be read over and over again. The principles will take time to affect change, so the idea is to read it and practice the contents often. Remember that losing weight is a long-term goal that will take time, patience, and discipline. You will feel better almost immediately once you start reading this book, though, and find that there are more than 200 pieces of valuable information that will help you reach your weight-loss goal.

Use the simple principles in this book as you would tools in a tool box. Refer to them as often as you need to. Flip to a certain page when confronted with that particular situation. For example, if you find yourself standing in the kitchen at 3 a.m., craving ice cream, flip to the simple principles that deal with how to avoid late night and emotional eating. Similarly, if you find yourself at a restaurant, unsure of how to stick to your diet, flip to the *Dining Out* chapter for suggestions that will help you make dining out a pleasant and dietetic experience. Above all, use it to adopt the habits, tricks, and practices that will allow you to successfully lose weight!

SETTING GOALS

The reasons people want to lose weight are as varied as the sizes and shapes we all come in. Some people want to lose weight for health reasons; others want to drop pounds to look more attractive. Those in the entertainment or sales industries must lose weight for career reasons, and there are even those who want to lose weight to meet a certain physical challenge, such as running a marathon or completing an endurance hike.

Regardless of why you want to lose weight, successful weight loss is almost entirely dependent on one important factor: setting realistic and sensible goals for yourself.

Studies consistently show that setting goals and reaching them is one of the most significant ways to achieve results, no matter what you are attempting. When you set your goals too high, you set yourself up for failure. For example, let's say in early April you decide to lose 15 pounds for your high school reunion scheduled for the end of that month. It is almost impossible to accomplish this goal in that amount of time, and absolutely impossible to do it in a healthy manner. But let's say in April you vow to lose 15 pounds by Christmas. This is a realistic goal you can reach with proper planning.

Defining realistic goals for your weight loss is important for a second reason: it will protect you against diet scams that waste your money and even endanger your health. Knowing what is realistic will allow you to avoid products and programs that promise too-good-to-be-true results. Similarly, avoid products and programs that promise significant weight loss without asking you to change your lifestyle. It is not realistic to lose weight without exercising or taking in fewer calories, so such a promise should be a red flag warning you to walk away from it. In addition to offering false hope, such products can be very dangerous. Indeed, misuse of diet pills has been proven to cause abdominal pain, nausea, pulmonary hypertension, insomnia, and heart disease. The following principles will help you determine what goals are realistic and will keep you both safe and motivated as you work toward losing weight.

PRINCIPLE #1

Identify your ideal weight.

—— ✳ ——

The most common reason people lose interest in their weight loss program is due to unrealistic goals. We can modify some aspects of our appearance through diet and exercise, but the rest is the result of genetics. Media images of the "ideal body" make us want the same type of figure for ourselves. When we are unable to reach this goal, we feel as though we have failed. View these images from a realistic perspective. Most people are not genetically predisposed to look like fashion models or superheroes. When you let go of unattainable ideals and focus on your own weight-loss potential, the pressure and stress related to weight loss can be relieved and better results can be achieved.

Principle #2

Expect to lose weight over time.

Weight loss is not instantaneous. Moreover, it's likely that the weight you want to lose has crept on over the years. Weight gain happens over time, through gradual overeating and lack of exercise. Weight loss will happen at the same pace, through slowly modifying your eating patterns and incorporating exercise into your daily routine. Use your common sense when it comes to losing weight. Weight loss that is healthy and has a chance of becoming permanent will happen at a steady rate. Reduce your calories by 250-500 calories a day and include at least 30 minutes of physical activity a week. Studies show that maintainable weight loss happens at a rate of 1-2 pounds a week.

PRINCIPLE #3

Figure out the factors that determine your weight.

Identify all the factors that affect your weight. This will give you an idea of the behaviors or conditions that you need to address to lose weight. Your current weight is the result of the following factors: your biology; your age and health status; the type and quantity of food you eat; the amount of physical activity you participate in; and whether or not you use food to satisfy needs other than hunger. Place extra effort into modifying the factors that you can control. Don't waste time and energy trying to change aspects of your appearance that are determined by age, genetics, or body type.

Principle #4

Adopt healthy habits at a slow pace.

Find out what your needs are in terms of food, nutrients, and exercise. If you have eaten freely and have been sedentary most of your life, you will need to change your diet gradually and include exercise at a reasonable rate. Adapting healthy habits at a slow pace will prevent you from being overwhelmed with change. For those who are already active and eat healthily, making additional changes to lose weight can be easier to accomplish. However, those who currently abide by an unhealthy routine will have to find more creative ways to modify their diet to enable them to lose weight.

PRINCIPLE #5

Know how your age affects the rate at which you lose weight.

———————— ✳ ————————

Understand the benefits and challenges of weight loss based on your age. During the 20's, this is the time to establish good habits. Studies show that people who have been active since their 20's have less fat when they reach mid-life versus those who have not made a point to eat healthy and exercise. During the 30's, it's easy to let pounds sneak on. Maintain a balanced body composition and fight bone loss by building lean muscle tissue. For those mid-life and above, a slower metabolism and hormonal changes may make it difficult to lose weight. Don't eat more than you need to at this age and participate in exercise to burn more calories.

Principle #6

Modify your diet and exercise plan as you lose weight.

The rate at which you lose weight depends on your current weight and the number of pounds you want to lose. Someone looking to shed 50 pounds may lose weight at a faster rate initially than someone trying to get rid of the last five pounds. Pounds are easier to drop if you have more to lose. As you lose weight, your body actually needs less calories to maintain itself. If you stick with the same program that you started out with, your weight loss will eventually plateau because your body has adapted. When your progress starts to slow down and you stop seeing results, modify your diet and exercise program.

PRINCIPLE #7

Focus on both short term and long term goals.

No matter how much weight you have to lose, your progress will be easier if you set up both short and long term goals. Make your weight-loss goals specific and attainable. Breaking down your program into smaller, more focused intervals will make these goals seem within your reach. Short-term goals will allow you to witness the more immediate results of your hard work. You will be able to build on these short-term successes and make realistic steps toward your final goal. Since weight loss takes time, it's important to track your progress through small measurements. Eventually, your long-term goal will be within your sight.

Principle #8

Aim for losing a pound a week.

Experts recommend that you lose a pound a week on a healthy weight-loss program. To lose a pound a week, you need to reduce your current caloric intake by 500 calories a day. This can be accomplished by working out to burn additional calories and modifying your diet to reduce the number of calories you eat. If you have lost weight initially but now have stalled, you probably have hit a plateau. Reassess your diet and exercise program and make sure you have not fallen back on old habits. Your body will resist dipping below a healthy weight. If you are slim and can't shed additional weight, you may have reached your body's target weight.

Principle #9

Calculate your daily calorie allowance.

Figure out how many calories your body needs. To calculate your daily calorie allowance, refer to page 269. The minimum calorie count you need to survive is called your Basal Metabolic Rate (BMR). You will also need to take into account the extra calories you expend based on your activity level. Your BMR, plus the number of calories you burn performing daily activities, is the total amount of calories your body needs to maintain your current weight. To lose weight, you will need to eat fewer calories or burn more calories than the amount of calories your body currently needs.

Principle #10

Create a calorie deficit.

Decide what foods to eat so you create a calorie deficit. A calorie deficit is the difference between the amount of calories your body expends versus the number of calories you consume. If the average person needs 2,000 calories to maintain their weight, then reducing their caloric intake to 1,500 a day would result in a 500 calorie deficit. This deficit would result in weight loss of a pound a week. You can still indulge in some of your favorite foods and lose weight as long as you maintain a calorie deficit. For example, balance out a high calorie breakfast by eating a moderate lunch and dinner.

Principle #11

Find out how many calories are in your favorite foods.

Check the calorie content and nutritional information for your favorite foods. A classic steak fajita dinner can contain more than 1,000 calories and 50 grams of fat. It's easy to see how people gain weight if they eat meals like this on a regular basis. Figure out the high-calorie foods you can eliminate from your diet. Find healthy, lower calorie substitutions to help you lose weight. Packaged foods require a Nutrition Label that indicates the amount of calories per serving. Many restaurants, take-out, and fast food places post nutritional information on line. There are also books and websites that will help you calculate the calories contained in specific foods.

PRINCIPLE #12

Consider the long term.

Frequent workouts and restrictive diets will enable someone to drop pounds quickly. However, this level of discipline will be difficult to keep up with in the long run. Studies show that to lose weight and keep it off, you need to modify your behavior in ways you can live with for years, not weeks. Make simple changes that you can practice over time to lose weight at a steady, safe, and healthy rate. You will gradually experience satisfaction, not only as you become lighter, but as your health, energy, and attitude improves. Rather than thinking of short cuts to temporarily shed pounds, focus on the long-term ways you can lose weight and keep it off.

Creating a
Weight Loss Plan

It is often said that those who fail to plan, plan to fail. Indeed, there is no surer way to sabotage your dream of losing weight than to neglect to enact a solid weight-loss plan. Coming up with a plan of action for your weight loss is one of the most important things you will do as you embark on the path to a thinner you. Your plans for weight loss should target three main areas; your food supply, exercise routine, and attitude.

First and foremost, you will need to develop a road map for what you will eat. Although this may seem simple, it actually takes careful planning. It is not likely that at the last minute you will throw together a meal that is well-balanced, nutritious, and also low in fat, high in fiber, and stays within your daily caloric limits. Take the time to plan out meals in advance. Make Tuesday night vegetable lasagna night; make Wednesday lunches feature Greek salads. Getting into a routine with your meals ensures you will stick to your dietary guidelines.

You must also plan an exercise routine and stick to it. Treat your weekly gym time as an appointment that cannot be rescheduled. Learn to view your morning walk as part and parcel of your day, such as brushing your teeth or reading the mail. Many of us tend to skip exercise because we feel we lack time for it. If this applies to you, learn to build time into your daily schedule to exercise; consider incorporating exercise into things you already have to do, such as cleaning the house or mowing the lawn.

Finally, planning for weight loss means mentally preparing yourself for the challenges that lay ahead. Losing weight takes effort, and you must be prepared to overcome temptation and laziness on a daily basis. You must shift your perception of dieting from a daunting, unpleasant chore to a healthy, invigorating activity. You must also be ready to prioritize your diet and choose it above other activities. This may mean occasionally missing out on social activities that involve drinking or eating if you think it will derail your progress.

Use the following principles to craft a course of action that will make your diet fit seamlessly into your daily routine.

PRINCIPLE #13

Change the way you look at diets.

The right attitude is important when losing weight. Look at dieting not just as a way to lose weight but as a healthy way of life. If you consider dieting to be merely a means to an end, eating the right foods will be difficult to maintain after you reach your goal. Without adjusting the attitude in which you look at dieting, it will be too easy to ditch the "temporary fix" you have adopted once you reach your target weight. However, reverting back to previous habits will only result in weight gain. Disassociate dieting with restriction and deprivation. Look at dieting as eating the right foods in the right amounts.

PRINCIPLE #14

Choose your diet plan carefully.

— ✳ —

Create a diet plan that is tailored to your lifestyle and personal preferences. There are many diet programs in the market. Make sure the program you choose focuses on realistic and achievable goals. Figure out the rate at which you expect to lose weight and the amount of time it will take to reach your goal. Research the credentials of any professionals involved with the program. Make sure the diet includes foods you enjoy, yet are low in calories and fulfill your daily nutritional requirements. A good program should also address how to keep weight off. Finally, consider the total cost for fees, packaged foods, and any other required items.

Principle #15

Be committed to losing weight.

---※---

Those who have lost weight and have kept it off state that a large part of their success was due to their commitment and mental preparation for the challenge. Before you start a weight loss plan, make sure you are willing to commit the time, energy, and expense involved in the process. Figure out if this is the best time to commit to weight loss. Determine if there are any external factors such as stress, financial worries, health, or physical concerns that may hinder your weight loss. Address these issues first. Then ask yourself if you are dedicated to changing your eating habits, exercising regularly, controlling your food choices, and preparing your own meals.

PRINCIPLE #16

Make losing weight a priority.

❋

Decide how important it is for you to lose weight. Prioritizing your weight loss will make it easier for you to choose options that will help you lose weight and avoid foods that may keep you from your goal. When ordering a latte, do you choose skim milk and skip the whip cream so you can reach your goal faster? Or would you rather go with the full-fat option and have the momentary pleasure of drinking something that tastes marginally better? Decide what changes you are willing to make to lose weight and stick with them. The gratification of gradual weight loss will be much more satisfying than the instant gratification of food.

Principle #17

Realize that losing weight takes effort.

It's easy to say "I'm going to lose weight." It's a bit more complicated to actually shed the pounds. It takes effort to lose weight and to keep it off. It's natural for the body to resist change. Survival means storing weight for protection in times of crisis. Your body tries to protect itself by slowing its "basal metabolism," the rate at which you burn calories while at rest. This makes weight loss harder. To counter this effect, it's important to make gradual changes in your eating habits. The people who succeed in losing weight have discipline. Successful dieters are diligent about sticking to their diet plan and make sure they meet their daily activity requirements.

Principle #18

Strive for consistency with your weight-loss program.

Weight loss will be easier to achieve and maintain if you are consistent with your approach to food. If you severely limit the amount and types of food you eat, you increase the chance that you will feel deprived. Deprivation generally leads to a cycle of starvation and bingeing. These extreme behaviors can actually make you gain weight. Try to include all healthy foods in moderation and eat your daily recommended amount of calories every day. If you happen to have an unplanned treat, don't give up your diet and overeat. And don't feel the need to overcompensate by starving yourself. Consistent behaviors will enable you to lose weight.

Principle #19

Take 30 days to try out something new.

Stick to any dietary and physical commitment for at least a 30-day trial period. After the first 30 days, you will have practiced the behavior long enough to consider it a habit. If you decide to continue, the commitment will be much easier to maintain. You'll also have broken any bad habits associated with the behavior. In addition, the success of sticking to the program for 30 days will encourage you to continue. You'll also have the insight from 30 days' worth of results. This feedback will help you make an informed decision for any long-term program. It will also give you an idea of what results to expect if you continue your weight-loss program.

Principle #20

Create good habits to reach your goal.

If you are trying to beat a bad habit, such as eating too much candy, replace it with a healthy habit. For example, instead of eating a candy bar, have a piece of fruit when you are in the mood for something sweet. Focus on including the good behavior into your routine every day for a month until it becomes second nature. Once you have established a good habit, try including another one. Work your way to the point where good choices are made automatically. Some examples of good habits to help you start out: go for a walk for 30 minutes a day instead of watching TV; have tea instead of soda; have a soup or salad and a smaller entree; order a sandwich with whole grain bread instead of white.

Principle #21

Seek expert advice.

Consider consulting a registered dietitian, or RD. He or she will be a highly trained food and nutrition expert who can help you with your weight-loss questions. Your doctor may also be able to determine if you have a physical condition or disease that has caused you to gain weight. Some disorders that can cause weight gain are low thyroid hormone, pituitary disorders, adrenal gland malfunctions, blood sugar imbalance, and fluid retention due to drugs, liver disease, or kidney disease. If you have specific dietary needs, such as diabetes or food allergies, or if you are a vegetarian, consult a dietetics professional on how you can safely lose weight and develop an appropriate eating plan.

Principle #22

Understand the type of diets available.

Gather information on the different types of diets you can choose from. Figure out the benefits and drawbacks of each plan. The following are typical types of diets on the market:

- **Fixed menu diet:** lists all the foods permissible on the diet.
- **Exchange type diet:** allows you to choose from a set number of servings from each food group.
- **Pre-packaged meal diet:** provides prepared meals in limited portions.
- **Formula diets:** substitute meals or snacks with a pre-mixed formula or food replacement bar.
- **Flexible diets:** suggest that dieters monitor the consumption of fat or calories to lose weight.
- **Fad diets:** promote fast easy weight loss through eating only specific foods and eliminating whole food groups.

Principle #23

Incorporate foods from each of the six main food groups into your diet plan.

There are six main food groups: grains, fruits, vegetables, dairy, meat/beans, and oils. Your diet should include foods from each of these groups for good health. Diets that omit entire food groups lack nutrients, vitamins, and minerals that are crucial when losing weight. Unhealthy weight loss occurs when dieters avoid entire food groups. When whole food groups are eliminated, you do not receive the balance of protein, carbohydrates, and plant-based nutrients that your body needs. Over an extended time, nutrient loss can lead to muscle deterioration, irritability, headaches, nausea, and severe health problems such as kidney and heart disease.

Principle #24

Follow basic nutritional guidelines to ensure you stay healthy while losing weight.

Create a diet that abides by the following guidelines to make sure that you are getting the proper nutrients. Get adequate vitamins and minerals by eating a wide variety of fruits and vegetables. Consider a supplement if your diet is low in calories. Eat at least 50–60 grams of protein to build and repair body tissue. Include a minimum of 100 grams of carbohydrates daily to avoid feeling fatigued or dehydrated. Make sure you get 20–30 grams of fiber to aid in digestion. Limit fat intake to no more than 30 percent of your total calories.

Principle #25

Make sure your diet plan includes enough calories.

If you maintain a diet that severely restricts calories for long periods of time, your body will have the tendency to go into "starvation mode," and your metabolism will slow down. During times of severe calorie restriction your body tends to store calories as fat and burn muscle as a way to conserve energy. You may also experience nausea, diarrhea, and fatigue. Drastically reducing the amount of calories you eat for extended periods of time can also lead to serious long-term health complications. Figure out your recommended caloric intake based on your age, weight, level of activity, and the rate at which you want to lose weight.

Principle #26

Don't rely on a weight-loss plan that completely eliminates carbohydrates.

Low-carb diets are difficult to maintain for prolonged periods of time because they severely restrict the foods we eat. Carbohydrates are crucial for losing weight as well as maintaining energy. Your brain only uses carbohydrates for fuel so it's important that you consume enough healthy carbs for your body to function at its peak. This nutrient provides us with energy as well as essential vitamins and minerals. Eliminating carbohydrates can also make you deficient of fiber, which can lead to gastrointestinal distress. At least 40 percent of your daily calorie allowance should come from complex carbohydrates found in fruits, vegetables, and whole grains.

Principle #27

Combine calorie reduction and increased activity to lose weight.

Incorporate a reduced-calorie diet with exercise to burn off fat. Both of these methods will result in a calorie deficit that enables your body to call on fat reserves for energy. Your rate of weight loss will depend on how many calories you burn through activity and the amount of food you eat. If you are currently reducing your calorie intake by 500 calories to lose a pound a week, you can lose even more weight by working out. Exercise to burn 500 calories three times a week and you will lose an extra half pound of fat a week.

Principle #28

Find weight-loss solutions that
do not involve crash dieting.

Crash dieting can have initial results but is not effective for long-term weight loss. The physiological effects of sudden weight loss can lead to additional weight gain after the dieters return to their typical habits. Losing weight rapidly on a crash diet is often the result of decreased muscle mass and water loss. Our bodies switch to fat storing mode if our weight decreases too quickly. When normal eating patterns are resumed after a crash diet, people tend to gain the weight back plus more. This is because the body's metabolic rate has slowed down and has been conditioned to store excess calories as fat.

Principle #29

Be wary of diet plans that sound too good to be true.

With over $40 million dollars in profit, the diet industry is constantly touting a new product as the solution to weight gain. With thousands of marketing dollars, these diets often promise you unbelievable results with little effort. Diets that rely on tricks are difficult to maintain and can damage your body. Learn how to distinguish a fad diet from a sensible one. Fad diets often exclude foods necessary for good health and do not instruct the dieter to build healthy eating habits. They are often too expensive to maintain for long periods of time. Fad diets use gimmicks to burn or restrict calories and make unrealistic statements like "miraculous, effortless, or instant weight loss."

Changing the Way
You Live

Many people do not realize that losing weight is just half the battle of weight loss. Focusing solely on losing weight is like driving somewhere but not knowing what to do once you arrive. You have made the journey and now need a plan of action. While many of us focus on simply losing weight, the key to successful weight loss is learning how to lose weight and keep it off. The most effective way to achieve this combination is to change the way you live.

As stated in the introduction, 98 percent of people who lose weight gain it back within five years. Perhaps even more astonishing, 90 percent gain back even more weight than they initially lost. Oprah Winfrey is one of the most high-profile people to have experienced the weight-loss weight-gain roller coaster. In the 1990s she became famous for losing an incredible 67 pounds—and then became even more famous for gaining more than 80 pounds back. Winfrey had lost weight but failed to change her lifestyle. She recognized this when she said in an interview with *People* magazine, "My greatest failure was in believing that the weight issue was just about weight."

Therefore, it is important to create a new lifestyle around the habits you used to lose weight in the first place. Institutionalize these habits into your everyday routine, creating a new way of living that will allow you to keep your lost weight off. The most effective weight-loss-friendly lifestyle changes you can make involve eating a balanced diet and exercising regularly. Consider your diet program as a foundation for how you should eat and exercise the rest of your life. If you go back to your old patterns, you will go back to your old weight. The healthy habits you learn as you lose weight should be permanently added to your lifestyle. These long-term changes can also lower your risk of certain diseases and improve your health and self-confidence.

Achieving a healthy lifestyle takes time, practice, and desire. Use the following principles to make small changes to your lifestyle that will help you lose weight and keep it off.

Principle #30

Make small changes to see big results.

Small changes can result in significant weight loss without drastically overhauling your daily routine. It takes 3,500 calories to make up a pound of fat. If a person saves 100 calories every day, they would save 36,500 calories in a year, or ten pounds of fat. If you save 500 calories a day, you can lose around a pound a week. Here are five examples of how you can save 100 calories in your day: jump rope for 8 minutes; chose low-fat turkey sausage instead of regular sausage for breakfast; order your sandwich without mayonnaise and cheese; take a brisk 15 minute walk; have water instead of soda with dinner.

PRINCIPLE #31

Splurge wisely.

Diets become overwhelming if you don't allow some flexibility. Give yourself a planned break every once in a while. Figure out what you can enjoy without undermining your weight loss. Be extremely picky with your splurge. You don't want to waste your treat on something you don't really enjoy eating. Or give up a day of exercise to sit back, relax, and spend some quality time with yourself. Spend a day at the park, have coffee with a friend, or read a book. Whatever you choose, select something that feels like a special break from your normal routine. You can then return to your program refreshed.

Principle #32

Give yourself enough time to burn off your evening meal.

Try to eat several hours before going to bed so your body has a chance to burn off extra calories. Most people are active during the day and sedentary at night. As a result, the least amount of energy is being used before bedtime. Eating huge amounts of calories at night, especially before going to sleep, creates an energy imbalance. You are providing your body with excess calories at a time when it needs them the least. Take a brisk walk after dinner, or do some chores, light exercising, or stretching to help burn off your evening meal.

Principle #33

Limit the number of carbohydrates you eat at night.

If you want to lose weight, consider eating fewer carbohydrates, such as white bread, chips, and cookies, before you go to bed. Researchers suggest that we are more likely to store fat when eating carbohydrate-rich foods at night. This is because the body doesn't handle insulin, the hormone that helps us process carbohydrates for energy, as effectively as it does in the daytime. As a result, calories from simple carbohydrates can end up being stored as fat. Replace high-carb snacks with protein, like a small yogurt, protein smoothie, or a small handful of nuts.

PRINCIPLE #34

Use sleep for recuperation instead of digestion.

Going to bed on a full stomach requires your body to expend energy on digesting food when it should be resting. The digestive system is not as effective while you are sleeping. This can cause heartburn, upset stomach, gas, bloating, while interrupting your sleep. It's important to allow your body to use sleep as time to recuperate from the day's activities. Sleep deprivation for a prolonged period of time can disrupt your body's natural ability to control weight. Lack of sleep can lead to an increase in appetite as well as cravings for fatty and sugary foods. Let your body recuperate at night by having a light evening meal.

PRINCIPLE #35

Have dinner three hours before going to bed.

Sleeping right after having a meal makes your body more likely to store excess calories as fat. During the night, our metabolism slows down and we burn fewer calories. Our bodies are focused on rebuilding our systems while we sleep, and our systems are reserving fuel for future use. During this storage mode, our bodies continue to expand by adding fat or muscle tissue. The problem is that the rate at which we burn calories decreases when we are asleep. If excess calories are consumed directly before bed, any undigested food ends up being stored mostly as fat.

Principle #36

Beware of trans fats.

Trans fats, or partially hydrogenated oils, disrupt your metabolism, cause weight gain, and increase your risk of disease. Experts have suggested that a diet high in trans fats can lead to weight gain even if the total number of calories consumed remains the same. In animal studies, evidence shows that trans fat also causes increased weight gain around the abdomen. Other risks include increasing low-density lipoprotein cholesterol (LDL, or "bad" cholesterol) and heart disease. Trans fats are found in nearly all packaged or commercially baked or processed foods. Avoid candy, chips, packaged snacks, pastries, donuts, cookies, and fried foods. When selecting foods, check the nutritional label for trans fat, hydrogenated, or partially hydrogenated oils.

Principle #37

Cut down on sugar.

America's sugar consumption has increased by 39 percent between 1950 and 2000. The use of added sweeteners has increased eightfold. Eat less sugar to effectively maintain your body's ability to burn fat. Large quantities of sugar can lead to weight gain because it is absorbed quickly into the system and causes elevated insulin levels, making you crave even more sugar. Large quantities of sugar also trigger your body to produce stress hormones that cause weight gain. Avoid high-fructose corn syrup, a simple sugar that is found in sweets and other processed foods like condiments, salad dressing, canned fruit, and soups. Check the sugar content on low-fat diet foods.

Principle #38

Shift in your seat.

Fidgeting and shifting around in your seat may seem like nervous habits. However, studies on posture allocation show that these seemingly insignificant movements can burn up to 350 calories a day. These additional calories amount to a weight loss of a pound every 10 days. This information is especially helpful for those with office jobs. Be aware of how you can move around when you are seated at your desk. Swing or bounce your legs, tap your feet or fingers. Alternate between flexing and relaxing your muscles or shift your weight from side to side. Occasionally get up and stretch. Take every opportunity to add movement to your day.

Principle #39

Read the label.

Always read the nutritional information for the foods you buy. If you have no idea what is in the food you eat, how are you supposed to know if it will help you lose weight? Learn how to read and interpret a nutrition label. Check out the Nutrition Facts label located on almost all packaged foods for the ingredient list. Pay extra attention to the serving size and number of calories, as well nutrients, portions, and percentage of daily nutritional values. Reading the label will help you select nutritious foods that are within your calorie limits. The label will also help you measure out correct serving sizes so you don't overeat.

Principle #40

Take a walk.

Moderately active individuals burn approximately 30 percent of their calories through daily non-exercise activity. Sedentary people only burn around 15 percent. Make a conscience choice to be more active every day. These activities are as simple as getting up in the morning, making breakfast, and driving to work. Add to these activities by parking farther away from your building; then, take the stairs or go for a walk during your break. There are endless ways to increase your overall activity level if you chose to do so. Move around whenever you get the chance; do chores around the house; walk briskly when shopping. Remember, if you are moving around, you are expending energy, burning calories, and losing weight.

PRINCIPLE #41

Get enough rest.

---------------------------------- ✳ ----------------------------------

Your body burns fat at an effective rate when you get eight
hours of rest. There is a crucial relationship between sleep
and the hormones that control your weight. A recent study
showed that lack of sleep increased levels of ghrelin, a hormone
that triggers appetite. It also showed decreased levels of
leptin, a hormone that enables the body to sense when it is
full. Past studies have also indicated a correlation between
inadequate sleep and increased body mass index. Sleep is one
of the most powerful states that enables your body to secrete
growth hormone. This chemical signals your body to utilize
fat for energy. The more growth hormone you secrete, the
more fat you burn.

Principle #42

Stay hydrated.

---------------------------- ❈ ----------------------------

There are many reasons why water is critical to the success of your weight loss program. Water is the main component of your body and is essential to function properly. Water enables your body to work effectively at burning stored fat. Proper hydration encourages and supports kidney function, which increases the liver's ability to process fat. Water can also help control the appetite. Often we think we are hungry when our body is sending us signals that we are actually thirsty or dehydrated. Drinking enough water also helps eliminate water retention and bloating. Aim for 64 ounces of water daily.

Principle #43

Eat low density, high volume foods.

Eating foods with high water content can help dieters by increasing the fullness factor. Research has indicated that on average, an individual consumes about the same weight of food each day. Typically, the weight of food eaten is more constant than the daily calorie intake. If the same weight of food is eaten, but the calories in each portion are lowered, fewer total calories will be consumed. Studies also showed that feelings of fullness did not change on lower calorie days. Fill up on low density, high volume foods such as fruits, vegetables, soups, stews, cooked grains, lean meats, fish, and lean poultry.

Principle #44

Ditch the sodas.

One 12–ounce serving of soda contains 140 calories and almost 40 grams of sweeteners, the equivalent of about 10 teaspoons of sugar. If you are drinking a soda with each meal, this can amount to 420 extra calories a day. Studies suggest that drinking sugar, especially the refined sugar found in soft drinks, can lead to weight gain even if you are not increasing your total daily calorie intake. Sugar in soda is quickly absorbed into the blood stream and is easily stored as fat. Sodas also create a spike in your blood sugar. This imbalance can lead to additional cravings. Replacing soda with water at mealtimes can help you lose around a pound a week.

Principle #45

Limit processed foods.

Diets high in processed foods have been linked to weight gain. Processing means that the components that are nutritious in healthy grains, such as wheat, rice, sugar cane and corn, are removed to make white flour, high fructose corn syrup, and simple white sugar. These refined carbohydrates are devoid of essential vitamins and minerals and are often high in calories. These foods are quickly digested and leave us feeling hungry shortly after eating them. Processed foods can also increase our appetite. Heavily processed foods, such as packaged snack foods, cakes, cookies, candies, and boxed meals, also contain high amounts of trans fats, artificial flavors, and preservatives, which impede weight loss.

PRINCIPLE #46

Decrease stress.

Stress can affect your weight loss in a number of ways. First, chronic stress can slow the rate at which you burn calories. As your metabolism slows, your body goes into fat storing mode. This can lead to weight gain even when you are eating the same amount of calories. Stressful situations can also increase cravings for salty, sugary snacks that are high in fat and calories. These comfort foods produce feel-good chemicals to counteract anxiety. Hormones produced under stress, such as cortisol and epinephrine, can lead to fat storage around the abdomen. Adopt some relaxation techniques such as yoga or deep breathing to reduce your stress levels and lose weight.

Principle #47

Choose carbohydrates wisely.

Complex carbohydrates found in whole grains, fruits, and vegetables may help you lose weight. These foods have high fiber content so they are digested slowly. Complex carbohydrates provide a low release of energy so your body has a greater chance to burn off calories before they get stored as fat. Complex carbohydrates are often higher in volume and lower in calories. It typically takes longer to eat a 100 calorie apple than it takes to drink a 100 calorie soda. Finally, these foods are more satisfying than their refined counterparts. The fiber and water in the apple will make you feel full, while the soda will be rapidly absorbed and leave you feeling hungry shortly after.

PRINCIPLE #48

Rethink snack foods.

We typically reach for familiar snacks like potato chips, nachos, pretzels, cookies, cakes, and candy. Limiting these foods to lose weight does not mean that you have to go without your mid-morning and afternoon snack. The trick is to choose the right foods. Having a small amount of food between meals can help you control your appetite, provides you with energy, and keeps your metabolism active. Packaged snack foods are often high in fat, sugar, and refined carbohydrates and are high in calories. Instead, have a satisfying snack that contains complex carbohydrates like whole grains, fruits, vegetables, low-fat dairy and lean protein. Keep the total calories between 100 to 200 calories.

PRINCIPLE #49

Keep the weight off.

The behavior patterns that help you lose weight are the same ones that will help you maintain your ideal weight. Studies show that less than a third of the people who lose weight are able to keep it off. Long-term success depends upon you making your new weight-loss habits a permanent part of your life. Studies indicate that dieters who have successfully maintained their weight loss: eat breakfast daily; weigh themselves once a week; watch 10 hours or less of TV a week; and exercise an hour a day. Maintain your weight loss by adopting a lifestyle that includes all foods in moderation, healthy alternatives to foods high in fat and calories, and daily activities.

PRINCIPLE #50

Eat at least 5 servings of fruits and vegetables per day.

Approximately 90 percent of Americans do not get the daily recommended servings of fruits and vegetables. Eating enough fruits and vegetables is one of the most important practices an individual can make to lose weight and maintain health. Fruits and vegetables have a high fiber and water content, which means they fill you up and keep you full longer. These foods are also low in calories compared to their volume. You can eat more of them and still keep your calorie consumption low. Fruits and vegetables also contain essential phytonutrients, vitamins, and antioxidants that are essential for good health.

Principle #51

Check food label claims.

Just because a product claims that it's "low-fat," "fat-free," "sugar-free," or "low carb" does not necessarily mean it will help you lose weight. "Reduced fat" foods contain 25 percent less fat than a regular brand. Foods labeled as "light" contain 50 percent less fat than the same regular product. "Low-fat" foods have less than 3 grams of fat per serving. Even if foods claim to have less fat or carbs, they might not be low in calories. Check the label to make sure the product does not contain extra sugar or fat. Products that are "reduced" often include other high calorie ingredients.

PRINCIPLE #52

Use smaller plates and bowls.

Control your portions and prevent overeating by using smaller dinnerware and flatware. Studies show that 70 percent of weight-loss test subjects were more satisfied with less food when their meal was served on a salad plate instead of a standard-sized dinner plate. Weight loss is about portion control. Make your meal seem like more food in proportion by serving it on smaller plates. Put away your 12" plates and switch to 8" ones instead. You'll end up eating less food. Using salad forks and teaspoons will enable you to eat more slowly. When you eat at a slower pace, you give yourself more time to recognize when you are full.

Principle #53

Serve your food hot.

According to researchers, increasing the temperature of foods can enhance our taste buds. Foods served hot can be more satiating so you are likely to eat less. The temperature of your meal can also influence how full you feel after you eat. When the temperature of your food is hot, you have to take time to eat it. It's difficult to scarf down large bites of very hot foods. Try to vary the temperature of the foods you eat. Serve yourself one hot food item if the rest of the meal is cold. Take the time to heat up leftovers or balance out a salad with some freshly grilled chicken.

PRINCIPLE #54

Pour drinks into taller, thinner glasses.

— ❋ —

If you pour drinks into short, wide glasses, chances are you serve yourself up to 30 percent more than you think. Calories can add up if you are drinking juice, alcoholic beverages, or soft drinks from these glasses. Switch to taller, narrow glasses to keep from drinking extra calories. People generally tend to think that a tall glass contains more liquid than a short, wide tumbler. Even if both glasses hold the same amount of liquid, the tall glass is perceived to have more. Also, studies have shown that calories from liquids are less satisfying, so it's good to limit the amount of calories you get from beverages.

STAYING MOTIVATED

If losing weight were easy, everyone would do it. Weight loss is a challenging, even daunting, endeavor, one that forces you to constantly monitor and push yourself. It is to be expected, then, that you will face periods where you feel fed up and unmotivated.

Times that are especially hard to stay motivated to stick with your diet are during holidays such as Thanksgiving, New Year's Eve, and birthdays. Such events are always accompanied by food, food, and more food. The desire to eat is overwhelming. We eat during the holidays because it is our primary method of celebrating. Food tends to be the glue that binds us together during our social gatherings. (Think how different your office holiday party or your aunt's New Year's Eve affair would be if there were no appetizer platters or desserts!) Eating during holidays is also driven by the inclination to not "miss out" on foods that are only served once a year, such as eggnog, stuffing, pumpkin pie, or birthday cake.

The best way to stay motivated during times of increased temptation is to give yourself permission to indulge in small quantities. Try to make it through Thanksgiving without overeating any of the delicious holiday dishes. Knowing that you can control your eating habits will go a long way to motivating you to stick with your diet. Focusing on the positive, taking one day at a time, and celebrating your successes are other excellent ways to build your willpower and keep you motivated toward your weight-loss goals. The following principles will arm you with other ideas for staying motivated during your most difficult dieting downturns.

Principle #55

Focus on the positive.

To stay motivated, focus on all of the good qualities you possess. Look forward to the improvements that losing weight will make to your physical and mental health. Positive thinking leads to action. These actions will help you progress toward your goal. Negative thinking leads to negative feelings and lack of motivation. Instead of fixating on all the "bad stuff," write down all of the physical qualities you like about yourself and the good things you have done for your body. Acknowledge your good qualities and tell yourself that you are making yourself even better by losing weight.

Principle #56

Define your incentive to lose weight.

---- ✳ ----

Improving your health, feeling better, and looking good are all typical reasons why people want to lose weight. Personalize your weight loss goal by coming up with an additional incentive that is specific to you. A great incentive can motivate you toward your goal. Schedule an event that you would like to lose weight for, such as your birthday, a vacation, or a high school reunion. Plot your weight loss goal toward this event. Make sure that you give yourself enough time to reach your target weight (allow 1-2 pounds a week). Maintain your weight loss and work to keep your weight the same the following year.

Principle #57

Take one step at a time.

———————— ✳ ————————

Studies show that it is difficult to maintain new behaviors if too many changes are made at the same time. If you jump into an extremely strict diet and rigorous exercise program all at once, it will be difficult for you to maintain these habits. Instead, choose a reasonable short-term goal and take on one component of weight loss at a time. Figure out your meal plan first. Once you become acclimated to your new foods, try incorporating some exercise. Once you feel comfortable at the gym, add in some weight training. Small measurable steps toward weight loss are often the most gratifying.

Principle #58

Track your progress.

Actively maintain a record of your starting point, progress, and results. Writing down the steps you take to lose weight will show how well you are doing. It will also indicate the effectiveness of your program. Start out by writing down your measurements and your starting weight. Make notes on your current health and fitness levels. Document changes to your weight, body size, energy and mood on a weekly and monthly basis. When you see concrete proof of your progress, you'll be a lot more motivated to stick with your program. Take before and after photos. There is no better way to visually track your progress.

PRINCIPLE #59

Watch your weight.

Weigh yourself regularly to track your progress. Some experts recommend that you weigh yourself once a week. More frequent weigh-ins can be discouraging if pounds do not drop as quickly as expected. Others suggest that weighing yourself everyday is the best way to maintain consistent weight loss and prevent pounds from creeping back on. Tracking your weight on a daily basis can help you keep a close eye on what eating patterns help you lose weight. If you step on the scale every day, be prepared to see your weight fluctuate by 1-3 pounds. Regardless of the frequency, weigh yourself at the same time of the day and with the same amount of clothes on or none at all.

Principle #60

Consider your resolution to lose weight as a benefit to yourself, not a test of your willpower.

Constantly pressuring yourself to be perfect can lead you to feel overwhelmed. This burden may cause you to revert back to unhealthy habits. Instead of viewing diets as a constant source of stress, consider losing weight as something good that you are doing for yourself. A positive outlook can help you make better food choices. Determine all the reasons why you want to lose weight. When faced with temptation, don't focus on the effort it takes to say "no." Instead, think of the benefits you can gain from sticking with your diet. Your decision to eat healthy will be easier.

Principle #61

Tell your friends and family.

Let the people in your life know that you have decided to lose weight. Even though you may be alone in losing weight, you won't feel alone if you ask for the encouragement and support of those around you. If you live with others, talk to them about the reasons why you want to lose weight so they understand your efforts. Tell them what kinds of foods you can eat and the foods you want to avoid. Tell them that you need to eat less and not to put pressure on you to keep eating. If you don't speak up, they may sabotage your diet without meaning to. Sharing your intentions creates a sense of accountability. Your healthy habits may inspire those around you to lose weight as well.

Principle #62

Join a weight-loss support group.

Share your experience with others who are working toward similar goals. Joining a weight-loss support group may help you stay motivated. Look for local or online communities where you can share your story, get weight-loss tips, and ask for advice. Let other members know when you succeed so they can share your happiness. Also let them know when things get difficult. Other members often have suggestions to help you get through tough times. In addition to being inspirational, these groups are also educational, give you a sense of accountability, and provide a sense of community.

Principle #63

Celebrate successes.

Celebrate your daily successes as well as your long-term achievements. Recognizing your effort and accomplishments will motivate you to continue with your weight-loss plan. Schedule rewards into your program to congratulate yourself for every positive step you make. Decide what constitutes a reward, such as losing five pounds or a week of both eating right and working out. Make your rewards healthy, non-food related, and appealing. Treat yourself to a massage, new workout gear, or a fun gadget. Tell yourself that each little success is a stepping-stone to your ultimate goal.

Principle #64

Be prepared for roadblocks.

You can do your best to prepare for circumstances that may derail your weight loss, but there are some occasions that may come as a surprise. There are times you may be tempted to deviate from your diet or workout routine. One day of indulgence will not jeopardize your hard work. Don't feel discouraged and abandon your program. Enjoy the splurge, but mentally prepare to go back to your routine the following day. Avoid being hard on yourself if you eat too much or skip a workout every once in a while. Just be sure not to repeat the same overindulgence and try to make up for it the following day.

PRINCIPLE #65

Do not confuse water loss with fat loss.

Approximately a quarter of all weight loss is water. Rapid weight loss of over 3 pounds a week is most likely due to the flushing out of large amounts of water. You may lose weight at this rate initially as your body releases impurities. However, this weight loss is short term. The most fat that an average healthy body can manage to lose is around two pounds a week. If you lose more than three pounds a week, you most likely are losing a combination of fat, muscle, and water weight. Low carbohydrate diets often cause the body to lose water weight in addition to fat.

PRINCIPLE #66

Realize that the last five pounds can be the most challenging to lose.

According to weight-loss experts and thousands of dieters, the final pounds are often the hardest to lose. Shedding the last five pounds requires shaking up your current program. At this point, good eating habits are probably second nature. Instead of following strict guidelines and paying close attention to every nuance of your diet, you may have allowed some variation that is hindering your goal weight. Initiate a new diet or exercise rule that will jump start your weight loss and follow your new rule very closely.

MAXIMIZING YOUR METABOLISM

We often hear about metabolism and its importance in helping us lose weight. But what exactly is metabolism, and how can you make yours work harder for you?

Metabolism is a series of chemical reactions that converts the food we eat into energy. This energy powers everything we do, from thinking to moving, healing, growing, and even aging. When people eat, they take in energy in the form of sugars (carbohydrates), proteins, and fats. But the body's cells cannot use energy in this form. So the body must break down these substances so the energy can be distributed to and used by the body's cells. Molecules in the digestive system called enzymes break down each substance differently: proteins are broken down into amino acids, fats are broken down into fatty acids, and carbohydrates are broken down into simple sugars, such as glucose. The process of breaking these substances down and using them for energy is called metabolism.

Metabolism is a very complicated chemical process, so it is easier to think of it in its most basic sense: metabolism is something that influences how easily you can gain and lose weight, or how easily you store or burn calories. The number of calories you are able to burn in a day depends on how high or low your metabolism is. Everyone burns calories at something called a basal metabolic rate, or BMR. This is the rate at which your body burns calories while at rest. Everyone has a different BMR, which in large part is inherited.

But you can actually change your BMR by doing certain activities and eating certain foods. For example, over time, regular exercise can increase your body's BMR. Adding more muscle to your body will also increase your BMR—muscle burns more calories than fat (about 6 calories per pound, versus 2 calories per pound). Finally, your eating habits— the time at which you eat and your intake of spicy or other metabolism-friendly foods—can increase your BMR. Use the following principles to make the most of your BMR and take your weight-loss program to the next level.

Principle #67

Eat breakfast.

❋

Men and women who eat breakfast in the mornings are far less likely to become obese than those who skip the most important meal of the day. Start your morning with a good breakfast and you will likely eat healthy foods throughout the day. Eating breakfast is essential for weight loss. Your body is deprived of food during the night, which causes your metabolism to slow down. If your cells don't receive sufficient nutrients post-fast, they will adapt and function less efficiently on smaller amounts of food. Skipping breakfast will actually train your body to store more fat when it senses you are not getting enough food.

Principle #68

Drink 5 cups of green tea daily.

※

Research shows that green tea can actually help you burn fat and increase your metabolism. Green tea contains very special compounds called catechin polyphenols. These antioxidants help you drop pounds by increasing fat oxidation and thermogenesis, the process where your body temperature increases as a result of burning fat. Green tea can also prevent the storage of excess sugar and fat in the body. Another antioxidant, epigallocatechin gallate (EGCG) has been shown effective at regulating glucose levels which may help reduce your appetite. Drinking 5 cups of green tea may burn 70-80 extra calories a day.

Principle #69

Eat spicy foods.

Some researchers suggest that spicy foods, primarily red pepper, cayenne, and chili pepper, may help raise your metabolism. These foods may increase your calorie burning capacity for up to 2-3 hours after eating. The heat generated from capsaicin can increase your body temperature and temporarily raise your metabolic rate by around 8 percent. While studies need to prove whether or not this rate has a profound effect on weight loss, eating spicy foods may also help you lose weight by increasing feelings of satisfaction. The additional water needed to quench the heat from foods may also aid in feeling full when eating a spicy meal.

Principle #70

Eat natural or whole foods.

The best foods for weight loss should be natural and should contain high amounts of nutrients and fiber. These foods should also be low in unhealthy fats, refined sugar, sodium, and calories. Create a healthy diet that focuses on unprocessed foods such as fruit, vegetables, whole grains, legumes (lentils, dry beans, and peas) and lean protein. Because fruits, vegetables, and whole grains are high in complex carbohydrates and fiber, they are digested slowly. The slow release of energy helps keep your blood sugar at a steady level and prevents cravings and surges in appetite. Dieters will find that they are able to eat more, consume fewer calories, and still satisfy their hunger when eating natural, or whole foods.

Principle #71

Add lean protein to your diet.

————————— ✳ —————————

Proteins are building blocks for your body. Unlike fat and carbohydrates, which are primarily sources of energy, proteins play an important role in the function and repair of body tissues. Proteins help build muscles and can increase your metabolic rate. It takes more energy for your body to digest protein than it does to digest carbohydrates or fat. This is because the increased "thermic" effect of digesting protein. The energy it takes to just digest and absorb protein accounts for approximately 25 percent of the total calories protein contains. Ground turkey, skinless white meat poultry, as well as egg whites, fish, and legumes are great sources of lean protein.

Principle #72

Increase your calorie-burning potential by eating small meals throughout the day.

Ensure that you are eating enough to keep your metabolism active. Increase your total calorie-burning capacity by having small, portion-controlled meals throughout the day. The act of eating helps increase your metabolism. The process of absorbing food requires energy. You burn calories with every meal as your body digests food. Keep your metabolism doing its job by spreading out large meals into smaller ones consumed throughout the day. You can end up burning more calories and still eat the same amount of food.

Principle #73

Eat at regular intervals.

Waiting too long between meals can slow down the rate at which you burn fat. Increase your metabolism by eating enough calories at regular intervals during the day. Try to have something small to eat every 2 to 3 hours. Avoid large gaps of time without food where your hunger completely takes over. If you skip meals your body starts conserving energy because it lacks nutrients. Instead of burning calories, your body starts to store them. Eating at regular intervals also aids in controlling hunger and prevents overeating later in the day when you are less likely to have time to burn off extra calories.

Principle #74

Burn more calories than you eat with nutrient, fiber-dense foods like fruits and vegetables.

Even though fruits and vegetables have calories, they are referred to as "negative calorie" foods. The digestive process requires more energy to utilize these foods versus the amount of calories these foods contain. Negative calorie foods usually contain high amounts of nutrients and fiber. The high fiber content requires more energy to digest than the amount of calories in the food itself. Some "negative calorie" foods you can eat are apples, asparagus, berries, broccoli, cucumbers, lettuce, grapefruit, oranges, melons, peaches, and plums.

Principle #75

Balance your energy levels.

Make sure your metabolism is working at it's maximum capacity so you can lose weight. Keep your metabolic rate active by balancing proper nutrition and exercise. Eat when your body will be most effective at utilizing food for fuel. Here are some tips to keep your energy levels steady. Eat first thing in the morning. Fuel yourself before a workout. Eating something light before you exercise will prevent your body from breaking down muscle tissue for energy. Eat soon after exercising to heal your body and restore energy. Having meals when you require energy will prevent you from eating large meals later when your body has little chance to burn off extra calories.

SECRETS FOR
PLANNING AHEAD

Our lives are packed with a multitude of commitments that take time and energy, and this also makes it difficult to lose weight. If we are late for an appointment around a mealtime, we tend to grab something packaged and unhealthy rather than something fresh and nutritious. If our errands take longer than we thought, we tend to skip the gym in favor of getting home to take care of more pressing things that need to be done. Indeed, work, school, errands, family, friends, and other daily tasks constantly threaten to derail us from working out and eating right. Unless we specifically plan to include healthy habits into our daily lives, the best laid dieting intentions often fall by the wayside.

Therefore, it is critical for the success of your diet that you don't leave healthy eating to chance. As Spanish writer Miguel de Cervantes Saavedra once wrote, "Forewarned, forearmed; to be prepared is half the victory." Prepping your meals in spite of a busy, stressful, or otherwise rushed day can make all the difference between a successful or a failed diet. Take the time to place healthy snacks at your desk or in your car. Familiarize yourself with locations along your route to work where you can make healthy "pit stops" if need be. Treat plans to exercise as appointments that cannot be rescheduled.

Dieting is hard enough; without the proper planning, your food and fitness choices will be infinitely more difficult to make. Use the following principles to incorporate your food and fitness priorities into your schedule the same way you would schedule a dentist appointment or job interview. View your dieting program as a schedule that must be kept. This may take time and discipline on your part. However, when faced with a tempting situation, use the following principles to help guide your decision toward eating healthy and losing weight.

Principle #76

Shop for groceries when you are not hungry.

Grocery stores use merchandising tricks such as smell, product placement, overall store layout, and sale items to get you to buy more. These ploys encourage you to shop longer and spend more money. You may end up buying more food than you need, especially if you are hungry. Stop by the grocery store after a large meal when you won't be as likely to stray from your shopping list. Or, drink a large glass of water beforehand. The feeling of fullness will make it easier to resist food not included in your program. Another tip is to chew on a piece of peppermint gum while you shop. You will be less likely to try free samples if your mouth is already occupied.

Principle #77

Navigate stores with efficiency.

Grocery stores are laid out to increase the amount of time you need to pick up basic items. The farther you walk inside the store, the more likely you are to see something that you want but don't need. Stores are designed to increase the time it takes to locate items. Staples like milk and bread are merchandised so you have to walk the entire floor to reach them. Become familiar with your grocer's floor plan and only visit the aisles that you need. Navigate the periphery of the store where fresh meat, fish, and produce are stocked. Avoid the aisles with the most tempting foods such as chips, cookies, candy, and pastries.

Principle #78

Make a shopping list and stick to it.

Focus on only the items you need to lose weight and stick with the items you have pre-selected as part of your diet program. Grocery stores stock the most tempting foods at eye level. It's easy to be side tracked if you let your eyes wander. It's also hard to resist a good bargain. Sale items can be difficult to pass up. Only consider items that you would normally include in your diet and don't get distracted by foods that are high in fat and calories or are overly processed. Making sure you have all the items on your list will make you less susceptible to bright packaging, enticing deals, and other impulse items.

Principle #79

Resist last minute temptations when you check out.

Check-out aisles are laden with foods that are high in fat, calories, sugar, and salt. Stores know that consumers waiting to pay for their groceries are a captive audience for these last minute "point of purchase" items. Avoid extra temptation by scheduling your grocery shopping when stores are not busy. Stores are most crowded right after work and on the weekends. Off peak hours include late night and early morning. Check out lanes will probably be bare during these times, enabling you to get in and out as quickly as possible.

Principle #80

Cook and eat meals at home.

———— ✳ ————

Prepare your own meals as often as you can. You can control exactly what goes into each meal if you make it yourself. There are many ways a seemingly healthy choice can be laden with hidden calories when not prepared by your own hand. Restaurant dishes, fast food, and take-out places can use preparation techniques, sauces, added butter, and fat that increase the calorie content without you realizing it. Also, the dishes include much more food than you would normally need. Meals made at home are healthier, and you can control how much you make and eat.

PRINCIPLE #81

Take note of the foods you eat and drink every day.

※

Jot down everything you eat and drink for several days to find out where all of your calories are coming from. Writing down every bite of food makes you much more aware of the type and amount of food you eat. Monitoring the food you eat regularly enables you to select healthier alternatives. Do you frequently eat candy? You may find that a piece of fruit can satisfy a sweet tooth. This research will help you determine the times you are likely to overeat and the foods that trigger you to overeat. Identify bad habits and turn them into good ones.

Principle #82

Don't rule out foods because of the time of day.

Try eating breakfast foods like eggs or steel cut oats as meals or snacks throughout the day. You'll have a lot more healthy options if you break the habit of eating certain foods only at a specific time of day. A hard-boiled egg with a bowl of oatmeal or whole grain cereal with skim milk can be great mid-afternoon snacks. These foods include complex carbohydrates, protein, and fiber to give you the boost of energy you need when your body is slowing down. If you don't have time to sit down for breakfast, make a turkey sandwich with whole grain bread and veggies. Eat half in the morning and save the other half for lunch.

PRINCIPLE #83

Be specific when planning your diet.

It's easy to say, "I won't eat junk food." But make specific modifications, so you don't fall back into old habits. Know exactly what you will eat when you have a craving for something salty or sweet. Instead of simply swearing off chips, cookies, cake, or candy, find healthy alternatives and have them available when you feel like snacking. For example, if your afternoon snack has consisted of a large personal bag of chips (300 calories) and a bag of Skittles (250 calories), have low-fat soy crisps (120 calories) and a medium apple (72 calories) instead. These options will save you over 350 calories a day!

Principle #84

Stock your freezer with healthy frozen entrees.

Look for entrees with protein, vegetables, and whole grains. They contain less fat, sodium, and preservatives than traditional frozen meals. Healthy Choice and Lean Cuisine are good options. Amy's Kitchen also supplies natural and organic frozen dishes. If you had a busy day, grab one from the freezer so you don't fall back on bad eating habits. Frozen entrees are portion controlled so you know exactly how much to eat. Each package also indicates the fat, carbs, protein, and the number of calories in each meal. Select entrees that range from 200 to 400 calories with less than 10 grams of fat.

Principle #85

Plan each week ahead of time.

Use your weekend to plan your menu for the following week. If you plan ahead on Saturday or Sunday, you are already in the mind-set to lose weight. And, you may be less likely to use the weekend as an excuse to overindulge. Figure out what your schedule looks like for the following week and stock up on healthy options. Decide what you want to eat and make sure you purchase ingredients to prepare meals. If you like to cook on the weekends, make extra so you can store and freeze leftovers in individual containers. Take these with you for an easy lunch option or re-heat one for a quick dinner.

Principle #86

Prepare your own meals in advance.

---- ❋ ----

It's hard to take time to cook a balanced meal or find a healthy snack if you are starving. It's much easier to eat whatever is the most convenient. If you prepare meals and snacks ahead of time you can make sure that a healthy option is always available. Have a yogurt smoothie for breakfast on a busy morning. When cooking fish or chicken for dinner, add a couple of extra pieces and use them in salads the next day. Make your own trail mix using dried fruit, nuts, and high fiber cereal and place single servings in resealable bags.

PRINCIPLE #87

Keep healthy staples in the fridge.

————————— ✳ —————————

You won't need to rely on take-out, fast food, or delivery if your kitchen is stocked with nutritious foods that are easy to prepare. Have the following basic items available at all times to lose weight: fresh chicken and fish; a variety of fruits and vegetables that can be eaten easily, such as baby carrots and celery sticks; apples, strawberries, and grapes; bagged lettuce for salads; low-fat milk and yogurt; eggs or an egg substitute; whole grain breads and high fiber/low sugar cereal; almonds or nut butters. If you keep these items on hand, you will more than likely eat them before they spoil rather than ordering something unhealthy.

Principle #88

Plan a healthy treat.

Include a healthy treat into your weight-loss plan so you don't feel deprived. Since it's easy to go overboard with sweet and fatty foods, choose items that are portion controlled. Treats should include some protein, fiber, and good fats. Try to keep these foods between 200 and 250 calories. There are many protein bars with decadent flavors such as mint chocolate and key lime pie. Make a strawberry shortcake using a high fiber waffle, a small container of light vanilla yogurt, and sliced strawberries. Other savory snacks include low-fat string cheese or high fiber crackers with hummus.

Principle #89

Keep a list of healthy foods, snacks, and meals you enjoy.

Make a list of all the foods you like that fit within your diet program. Many people feel like they have nothing to eat when they are losing weight. Planning meals is difficult if you don't know the foods that are available which fit in your diet program. If you write down all the foods you can still include in your diet, your options seem a lot wider and more appealing. Consider different foods for breakfast, lunch, dinner and snacks. Make a list of five to seven different options that you like for each mealtime. When planning ahead, this will give you more freedom and variety to choose from.

Principle #90

Find ways to stick to your diet when you are stuck on an airplane.

If you are spending a lot of time in airports and on planes, it's best to have a strategy that enables you to still lose weight. Have portable, healthy snacks on hand when you are caught with delays or are faced with the in-flight meal. The average airline meal can contain approximately 700–1000 calories and is filled with excess fat, sodium, and calories. The typical airline snack pack does not fare better, containing up to 450–800 calories of processed foods. Ward off extra calories by packing your own snacks of raw, pre-cut veggies, dried fruits, nuts, and whole wheat crackers with natural peanut butter.

Principle #91

Create a dietary itinerary to lose weight while traveling.

Losing weight while traveling is possible if you address situations that may derail your diet in advance. Create a schedule so you have healthy options at all stages of your trip. First, have something healthy to eat before you leave. Then you will be able to bypass the tempting airport food court without your appetite kicking in. Pack some light snacks in case you get delayed. Upon arrival, look up healthy restaurants in the area or ask the concierge if they have some recommendations of restaurants that are "diet friendly." It's easy to let calories slip by when traveling, so be vigilant and reduce your total calorie intake whenever possible.

Principle #92

Keep some meal replacement options in your car and at work.

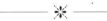

There will be circumstances out of your control where eating a fresh meal will not be possible. Rather than relying on fast food or snacking from a vending machine, have some non-perishable emergency meals handy in your car and at work so you can stick to your diet. Meal replacement shakes and bars are great for people with hectic schedules. Beware of bars containing too much sugar and fat. Healthful options contain a good balance of protein, fat, and carbohydrates. Look for bars or shakes that contain no more than 5-7 grams of fat, at least 3-5 grams of fiber, around 15 grams of protein, and 35 percent of your daily allowance of vitamins and minerals.

Curbing Your Appetite

Our need for food is first and foremost a biological need. Our body needs calories, fat, nutrients, vitamins, carbohydrates, water, and proteins to carry out complex biochemical reactions that allow us to grow, heal, and function. But of course, if eating were primarily about giving our bodies the energy they need to function, we would simply take a pill or gel that contained our daily nutritional values and call it a day. In reality, eating in our culture is a social activity often dictated by our appetites for certain kinds of food.

This love of food, or what we call our "appetite," however, causes us to eat when we are not hungry; to overeat because we like how a food tastes; to crave foods that are bad for us; and to substitute eating for other activities when we are bored or restless. Our love of eating causes us to forget the primary biological reasons we are supposed to eat. This combined with technological advances in food preparation and preservation, and a higher standard of living, provides us with a dizzying array of choices through which to satisfy our hungry stomachs.

Controlling your appetite is clearly an important step to take while dieting. The best way to curb your appetite is to continually remind yourself that while eating is pleasurable, you should do so first and foremost because you have a biological need to eat. The following principles will help you restrict your desire for food when your body does not really need it. Incorporate each idea into your diet program to minimize the amount of needless overeating you do each day.

Principle #93

Identify your hunger.

The key to losing weight and preventing weight gain is to identify your hunger and find ways to satisfy it in a healthy manner. People have a hard time losing weight because they eat when they are not hungry. And they overeat when they are extremely hungry. Sometimes they feel hungrier when they eat certain foods. Since you cannot avoid food, you need to identify your hunger and find a way to address that need in the right way. Figure out if you are experiencing true physical hunger, low blood sugar hunger, cravings, comfort eating, or social hunger. Find reasonable ways to deal with each situation.

Principle #94

Know what foods trigger your appetite.

---- ✳ ----

Identify the foods that send your appetite out of control. These are foods that you find yourself compulsively overeating after one bite. Common trigger foods usually combine sugar and fat, or fat and salt. Binges are linked to the food itself. For example, if donuts are a trigger food, a single bite can result in a person eating an entire box of donuts regardless of the person's hunger, situation, or emotional state. While experts say to eat all foods in moderation, it may benefit some people to avoid their trigger foods until they are able control these impulses. Try limiting these foods or avoid them altogether.

Principle #95

Find ways to control your hunger.

※

People often think that they have to go hungry to lose weight. You can still feel satisfied, have foods you enjoy, and eat fewer calories. The trick is to control your hunger. Keep your appetite stable by choosing lower calorie, nutrient dense foods, such as apples, sweet potatoes, salads, and grilled chicken. These foods will fill you up and still promote weight loss. Also, break up your meals and eat smaller portions at regular intervals throughout the day. By eating smaller meals more frequently, you will practice portion control and never feel like you are starving.

PRINCIPLE #96

Don't eat if you are not hungry.

Our bodies are conditioned to expect food at specific times of the day. If your routine has consisted of three large meals a day, it may be challenging to adjust to smaller quantities and different eating patterns. Your previous routine can also urge you to eat even if you are not hungry. If you had a late lunch at four, your body will still want dinner at six out of habit. Slowly adjust the frequency and quantity of your meals. Instead of having a full dinner after eating a late lunch, have a small snack such as a bowl of soup or an apple with a teaspoon of peanut butter.

Principle #97

Realize that seeing foods you crave can make you want to eat them more.

―――――――――――――― ✳ ――――――――――――――

Your sense of sight is a key factor in controlling your appetite and losing weight. Research has shown that brain waves are very different when people look at foods they like versus foods that they don't like. Even a photo of a tasty dish can increase your appetite. Don't linger over menus with large images of high calorie platters and desserts. Also, don't let your gaze wander to other dinners when eating out. Simply recognizing that sight has a significant impact on your appetite will help you fight the temptation to eat when you are not hungry.

Principle #98

Pass on dessert.

Even when we are stuffed, it can be hard to pass up dessert. The habit of eating dessert can make us expect something sweet at the end of a meal. The desire for sweet flavors has not been satisfied from the meal, so we eat something afterward to fulfill this craving. Add a little bit of sweetness to your main meal to prevent a craving for dessert. Sometimes a bit of apple or cranberries in a salad or a fruit sauce on fish or chicken can help you steer clear of the dessert menu. If you must indulge, try to minimize the damage with fresh berries and whipped cream.

Principle #99

Steer clear of refined carbohydrates.

———————————— ✳ ————————————

People who eat large, heavy meals with white pasta, rice, bread, or pastries and donuts may feel hungry again within a short time. Even though they have consumed a large quantity of food, refined carbohydrates digest very quickly and cause extreme fluctuations in blood sugar levels. These carbohydrates cause blood sugar to spike and drop. When blood sugar is low, our body produces feelings of hunger. This surge in appetite indicates that we need to consume more of these refined foods to increase our blood sugar level. Eat complex carbohydrates with the proper amounts of protein and fat to lose weight. These foods slow the digestion process and the release of sugar into the bloodstream.

Principle #100

Avoid alcohol.

Drinking too much may decrease your ability to burn fat as well as reduce your willpower and self control. Alcohol can lead your body to store fat. Your body processes alcohol first, before protein, fat, or carbohydrates. Drinking slows down your ability to burn off other calories. All the foods you eat while you drink are more likely to be stored as fat. Also, since alcohol is usually consumed in social settings where food is involved, drinking may lead you to overeat. As with any food, alcohol contains calories. If nothing else, eliminating alcohol will help you cut calories that have little nutritional value.

PRINCIPLE #101

Eat slowly.

---- ❉ ----

Eating slower may help people lose weight. Studies show that individuals end up eating less when they eat slower than their usual pace. Researchers state that subjects may have eaten less because they had enough time to feel satisfied and stopped eating. It takes up to 20 minutes for the brain to recognize that the stomach is full. During this time, it is very easy to stuff yourself with much more food than you really need. Use smaller utensils, take smaller bites, chew your food thoroughly, and put your utensil down between bites. Try eating half of what's on your plate, wait ten minutes, then have a few more bites if you're still hungry.

PRINCIPLE #102

Eat more fiber.

❄

Eating foods rich in soluble and insoluble fiber increases the feeling of fullness and slows the rate at which you digest your food. You can be satisfied with less food for a longer period of time without feeling hungry again. Studies also show that unrefined foods that are high in fiber such as fruits and vegetables and whole grains can stimulate appetite suppressing hormones. Research indicates that the average person can lose more weight if they increase their fiber intake to 25 grams per day. Studies show that people who increase their fiber consumption can lose up to 10 pounds in a year. Great sources of fiber include fruits, vegetables, beans, legumes and whole grains.

Principle #103

Brush your teeth after meals.

— ✳ —

Brushing your teeth after meals can help curb your appetite so you can lose weight. If you are having a hard time pulling yourself away from your meal, get up and brush your teeth. The flavor change may help keep you from eating more. If you can, keep a travel size toothbrush and toothpaste set with you. Store a set in your car and at work as well. If you don't have toothbrush and toothpaste handy, try a peppermint or chew a piece of gum to signal that the meal is over. Also, if you are susceptible to nighttime snacking, brush your teeth early so you won't be tempted to snack after dinner.

Principle #104

Refuel regularly to prevent overeating.

※

Eating small amounts of food throughout the day will guarantee that you never feel the extreme hunger that compels you to overeat. Let your body know it's going to get a satisfying amount of calories on a regular basis. If you starve yourself all day and then have dinner, you're probably going to eat much more than you need to before your brain tells you to stop. Lose weight by eating breakfast and having snacks that combine lean protein with complex carbohydrates. For example, have a piece of low-fat cheese with an apple or almond butter spread on whole-grain crackers between meals.

Principle #105

Never feel deprived.

Don't make your favorite foods off limits, because you will immediately crave what you deny yourself. Feelings of deprivation generally lead to overeating. Schedule a favorite food into your diet the same way you schedule exercise. Planning ahead allows you to balance out your indulgence by incorporating an additional workout or eating lightly the rest of the day. A typical ½ cup serving of full-fat ice cream is 280 calories and 15 grams of fat. It would take around one hour to walk off these calories. When you feel like having a high calorie food, ask yourself if it's worth the time it would take to burn it off.

PRINCIPLE #106

Know the difference between psychological and physical hunger.

※

Identify emotions, situations, or environments that cause you to overeat. It can be challenging to lose weight because not all hunger is based on the body's need for energy. Be able to tell the difference between the times you eat because you physically need to and the times you eat for psychological reasons. Sometimes the mere sight or smell of food entices you to eat. Emotions such as boredom, happiness, or anxiety are causes of psychological hunger. Eating a balanced meal should keep you satisfied for 3 to 4 hours. If you feel like eating when you are not physically hungry, find ways to distract yourself until the craving subsides.

Principle #107

Monitor your eating habits.

---❋---

Recognizing habits that cause you to overeat may help you lose weight. Over the years, we expect to eat at certain times of the day. We use food for celebration. Food becomes the source of comfort when we are feeling sad. We indulge in food when we are stressed and tired. Track your eating habits to find out where your extra calories are coming from. Find patterns that lead to overeating and address these issues. Do you have trigger foods? Do you eat when you are emotional, under stress, or when you have nothing else to do? Monitor your habits so you can avoid eating when you don't need to.

Principle #108

Listen to your body.

On a scale from one to ten, where 1 is starving, 5 is neutral, and 10 is stuffed, you should eat at the beginning stages of hunger (4) and stop when you are comfortably satisfied (6), but not past the point of being full. Do not let yourself go past the point of initial hunger. If you delay eating and allow yourself to get weak or fatigued (2), you may find that it's hard to stop eating once you've started. Do you overeat until you are uncomfortably full (8) or when there is unlimited food being served? Listen to your hunger signals to help you decide when and how much to eat.

Principle #109

Prevent emotional eating.

A research study on emotional eating suggests that dieters who address this issue are more capable of long-term weight loss maintenance than those who simply diet and/or exercise. Handling emotions without food is a technique that helps dieters lose weight and keep it off. There are four steps to prevent emotional eating. First, recognize the emotions that trigger you to overeat. Second, identify the situations that make you experience these emotions. Third, find alternate ways to deal with emotions, such as working out regularly or spending time with good friends. Last, build a support group that you can talk to when you feel the urge to overeat.

PRINCIPLE #110

Skip the variety pack.

————————————— ✳ —————————————

Too much variety can cause you to overeat. A study showed that participants ate almost 25 percent more food when offered foods containing three different flavors with distinctive texture and color than when they were presented a single flavor. Snack food companies have included an overwhelming number of options in their product lines. A leading snack manufacturer offers 150 different types of chips and a leading soda company produces over 400 soft drinks. With all the options available it's no surprise that snack foods are one of the most commonly overindulged foods. Enjoy a single serving of one snack at a time to lose weight. Pass on snack mixes that combine a variety of chips, pretzels, and nuts.

Principle #111

Be the last person to start eating when dining with others.

People tend to eat between 40 percent and 70 percent more food when eating with groups of seven or more people. We tend to adopt the eating behaviors of the majority, no matter how unhealthy they may be. Be the last to start eating in groups in order to lose weight and keep calories down. Also, recognize that the social interactions within groups of people tend to lengthen mealtimes. Longer mealtimes increase the likelihood that you will eat more. Don't feel the need to keep up with the table and match each bite of their food with your own. Leave the high calorie appetizers for the rest of the table to finish.

Controlling Your Portions

In 2005 a fascinating study about portion control was undertaken by the North American Association for the Study of Obesity. Researchers recruited 54 participants to take part in a study involving soup. Some of the participants were given a regular bowl containing a regular portion of soup and asked to eat as much of it as they liked. Other participants, however, were given a self-refilling bowl of soup. Soup was automatically piped into the bottom of the bowl as the participants were eating, making it impossible for them to ever reach the bottom. But the participants were not told that extra soup was being added to their portion; the soup was piped in so slowly it was impossible for the participants to tell that soup was being added as they were eating it.

Researchers found that participants who ate from the self-refilling bowl ate a whopping 73 percent more than did participants who ate from a normal bowl. Perhaps more astonishing was the fact that those who ate from the self-refilling bowls did not report feeling any more full than those who ate from the regular bowls. Furthermore, the study found that a person's weight did not affect whether they were likely to keep eating soup from the self-refilling bowls. Participants eating from the self-refilling bowls included both overweight, normal weight, and underweight participants. Across the board, everyone ate more, no matter what their weight or disposition.

The study was helpful in proving what many of us have already come to learn: that the size of your portion determines how much you will eat. To lose weight, therefore, you must control the size of your portions. Learn to become on guard for situations in which you may be served large portions or for environments in which you are likely to overeat. Use the following principles to learn habits, tips, and tricks to keep your portions reasonable and your diet on track.

Principle #112

Split your meal in half.

An easy way to cut calories and still eat your favorite foods is to divide your meal and only eat half. Substitute the other half with soup, fresh veggies, or a piece of fruit. If your typical dinner consists of two slices of pepperoni thick-crust pizza, replace the second piece of pizza with a garden salad and light dressing. This simple change can save you around 350 calories. Also, pre-determine how much food you will eat. Instead of eating directly from the pizza box, take a slice, wrap up the rest, and put it in the fridge. Doing this will help you keep your portion sizes moderate and prevent overeating.

Principle #113

Do not buy anything mega, super, or king sized.

Bigger is not always better, especially in relation to our waistline. Almost all individually sized chips, cookies, and candies come in extra large sizes. These packages, marketed for single consumption, can have an overwhelming amount of calories. A king size candy bar can pack up to 500 calories and 25 grams of fat. A large personal bag of crunchy cheese sticks can have around 525 calories and 33 grams of fat. These large sizes are usually 2 to 3 single servings. These snack bags have more calories and fat than a 6 oz sirloin steak and a small plain baked potato with steamed broccoli.

Principle #114

Order single items rather than combo or meal deals.

Fast food restaurants lure customers with "combo meals" that include a variety of items at a low price. Or they advertise deals like "Buy one, get one free." Avoid these marketing ploys no matter how great the value. The amount of calories in a single meal can contain more than a days worth of calories. For example, a ¼ pound cheese burger, large fries, and a 21 ounce milk shake has over 1,800 calories. If you have to eat fast food, you can still lose weight by creating your own combo. Order a single burger or grilled chicken sandwich with a salad. The kids menu also has much more reasonable portions.

PRINCIPLE #115

Figure out the serving size of your favorite foods.

Did you know that an individual serving of mini pretzels is 20 pieces or that 14 to 16 potato chips is considered a single serving? You may be surprised at what is the standard serving size for most foods. It's important to figure out serving sizes so you can control the amount of food you eat and the number of calories you consume. Check the nutrition label for serving sizes. If you have been eating much more than the standard, cut down your portions. Don't eat out of the container. Measure out amounts of foods based on serving sizes.

Principle #116

Learn to eyeball portion sizes.

Keep the following comparisons in mind when eating foods that are not labeled with specific serving sizes. Knowing these portion sizes will help you lose weight. A 3 ounce serving of meat or chicken is comparable to a deck of cards; a 3 ounce serving of fish should look like a checkbook; a 1/2 cup serving of potatoes, rice, or pasta is similar to half a baseball; an ounce of cheese is the size of your thumb. For fruits and vegetables, aim for 1 cup servings. This can include a medium piece of fruit, a baked potato the size of your fist, and salad greens or veggies the size of a baseball.

PRINCIPLE #117

Minimize your options.

Research shows that over the past decade, the daily caloric intake of the average American has increased by up to 350 calories. Experts believe this extra intake is due to the number of options we have to choose from. Studies show that when you eat a variety of foods rather than a single dish, you end up eating almost 40 percent more food. There is a mental process that makes the first bite of food taste very good and then progressively less so called sensory specific satiety. Eating a different type of food, even when you are full, can make you want to eat more until you are satisfied with that particular flavor. Limit your meals and snacks to one or two food items to keep calories down.

Principle #118

Purchase favorite foods in small packages or single-serving bags.

Having trouble measuring serving sizes? It may be easier to buy foods in single-serving packages. The snack food industry is getting wise to the fact that consumers want to eat healthier. As a result, companies are paying more attention to the way they package their products. Popular snack foods are now being packaged in 100 calorie pre-packs. You can still have a snack and lose weight as long as your portions are moderate. Eat a controlled amount from a single serving package instead of mindlessly eating from a large bag. Just make sure you don't eat more than a single bag in one sitting.

Principle #119

Divide your plate with protein, carbohydrates, and veggies.

A simple way to stick with moderate portions is to figure out the proportions of protein, carbohydrates, and vegetables for your meal. Divide your plate into halves to ensure you are getting the appropriate amount of food from each food group. Start out by filling the first half of your plate with non-starchy vegetables such as a salad, green beans, or grilled tomatoes. Fill a quarter of your plate with protein. Choose from fish, poultry, or lean cuts of beef. The other quarter should be a starchy vegetable or grain like sweet potatoes or brown rice.

Principle #120

Serve yourself a healthy portion then put the rest away.

It will be less tempting to serve yourself seconds if the food is no longer within reach. When food is in your immediate vicinity, the chances that you will eat it increase, even if you don't feel like eating and even if you are already full. Availability is one of the most common reasons for overeating and picking at foods when hunger is not an issue. Lose weight by keeping serving dishes in a separate room. Immediately place extra food in an opaque dish and store it in the refrigerator. Leftovers that have cooled off will be less tempting.

Choosing Healthy Alternatives

One tendency of the average American eater is to run in the other direction when they hear the word "healthy." Indeed, many people mistakenly think that foods that are healthy must necessarily be unsatisfying or taste bad. Of course, this isn't so. To lose weight and keep it off, it is important to change your perception that healthy foods will not satisfy you as much as your favorite dishes. In fact, many people find they actually prefer the taste, texture, and smell of healthy foods to higher calorie ones once they become familiar with them.

As a nation, we have been somewhat brainwashed to view reduced or low-fat foods as second-class to the original. But in many cases, reduced fat or low-cal foods are indistinguishable from their higher calorie counterparts. Sometimes, the low-fat version is actually tastier! In fact, many people—dieters and non-dieters alike—report enjoying the "mouth-feel" of certain low-fat foods, such as baked, rather than fried, potato chips. Indeed, baked chips have found enormous popularity in the marketplace because they deliver a satisfying crunch that is different—and in some opinions, better—than fried chips. For this reason, baked potato chips are bought by both dieters and non-dieters.

It is therefore important to discard the mind-set that reduced or low-fat food must automatically be a worse product than the original. Recognize that just because you learned to like the high-calorie version of a product does not mean it is actually better. It simply means you were exposed to this version first. So the next time you shop, try the reduced fat version of your favorite food. You might even find you like it better.

PRINCIPLE #121

Try reduced fat or low-fat options of your favorite foods.

Try the reduced, low, or fat free counterparts to your favorite foods. These will help reduce your total calorie consumption. Switch from whole milk to skim and save 60 calories a cup. Have a light yogurt with reduced fat and sugar and save 70 calories. Three ounces of reduced fat cheese has around 120 calories less than regular cheese. Check the label for the specific reductions in fat, sugar, and calories. If completely eliminating potato chips is too difficult, buy the baked kind and save 40 calories per serving. Simply finding an alternative can decrease the total number of calories you consume over time.

Principle #122

Have a bowl of soup.

Studies show that when water is added to vegetables, like in soup, the soup is more satisfying than when the vegetables are eaten alone with a glass of water. Soup is relatively low in calories per serving. The high water content in soup sends messages to your brain that you're full. Since soup is served hot, you can't eat too much too quickly. Bites are always a spoonful. Have a tomato-based soup with high-fiber whole grains, beans, vegetables, and/or lean meat to lose weight. The extra ingredients will take time to digest and leave you feeling full longer. Avoid cream-based soups since they contain butter and fat and are high in calories.

Principle #123

Substitute dark chocolate for milk chocolate.

At 230 calories for a typical 1.5 oz bar of milk chocolate, the extra calories from sugar and fat found in this common craving can quickly add up. There are some alternatives that are better for you and still satisfy a chocolate craving. Dark chocolate is a good alternative to milk chocolate. Dark versions are known to contain flavoniods. These are compounds that can actually help lower cholesterol and reduce your risk of heart disease. Since good dark chocolate has a very rich and intense flavor, a small square can satisfy your taste for chocolate more than a full size milk chocolate bar. Look for bars with at least 70 percent cacao content.

PRINCIPLE #124

Grill, bake, or broil instead of frying.

— ✳ —

Change the way you prepare foods to cut out excess calories. Frying instantly adds extra calories from fat. A gram of fat contains 9 calories while carbohydrates and protein contain 5 calories per gram. Five ounces of a roasted chicken breast contains 260 calories and 5 grams of fat. A battered, deep fried chicken breast can pack up 400 calories and 21 grams of fat. Try grilling, broiling, or baking your meats, chicken, and fish instead of frying them. The way you prepare your food can make a huge difference in how much weight you lose. You can also try sautéing foods or pan frying using a non-stick spray to reduce calories and fat from your diet.

Principle #125

Remove the skin from poultry to lower fat content.

Get rid of all the extra calories that sneak into your meals. With 25 grams of protein per serving, chicken and turkey are great sources of lean protein. To keep these protein sources lean, remove the skin before preparation. A 3 ounce serving of chicken with skin has twice as much fat as preparing it without. Poultry is the staple of many weight-loss diets, and can be prepared any number of ways. Chicken or turkey can be included in salads, soups, sandwiches, ground for low-fat burgers, or served with vegetables. The options are endless. Make sure that your preparation methods eliminate extra calories from otherwise healthy options.

PRINCIPLE #126

Add flavor when you reduce fat.

A lot of the flavor from unhealthy dishes comes from fat. When you take traditionally high-fat foods and just remove the fat, the dish may end up tasting bland. Either you end up eating more because you continually try to experience a flavor that can't satisfy or you end up reverting back to the full-fat option. Add spices to your food to make them more satisfying. For an easy addition of flavor, use all-purpose spice mixes such as Chinese five-spice, Jamaican, or Italian seasonings. If you still miss fat, use an olive oil spray for a dash of flavor so you can have flavor and still lose weight.

Principle #127

Satisfy your sweet tooth with comforting spices.

There are many ways you can satisfy a sweet tooth without cookies, cakes, candy, or ice cream. The urge for something sweet can often be satisfied when you add spices to certain foods. There are a variety of spices that we relate to homemade desserts. Vanilla, cinnamon, nutmeg, clove, ginger, and allspice are the typical spices added to pastries and sweet baked goods. Adding these flavors to other foods that are already naturally sweet, such as baked apples, pears, and sweet potatoes, are all good ways to achieve the flavor that we crave from baked goods without all the extra sugar, fat, and calories.

Principle #128

Modify your recipe with healthy ingredient substitutions.

There's no need to throw out your favorite recipes. Just find healthy substitutions for the high-calorie ingredients. Switch out some of the high-calorie ingredients with low-calorie substitutions to retain flavor and still reduce calories. The following are simple changes you can make to your recipes to lose weight. Use nonfat sour cream for sauces. Replace ground beef with ground chicken or turkey. If the recipe calls for butter, margarine, or shortening, use only half the amount and replace the other half with applesauce. Replace whole eggs with two egg whites and just a tiny bit of yolk. Use condensed skim milk for whole milk.

PRINCIPLE #129

Subscribe to healthy cooking and food magazines.

Buy a healthy cookbook or food magazine for great tasting recipes to lose weight. These resources often have the nutritional value of each recipe so you can easily keep track of calories in addition to the fat, carbohydrates, fiber, sugar, sodium, and protein content per serving. Many cooking websites have "healthy living" sections where the recipe is built with alternative ingredients. Experts have already found a combination of flavors and spices that make the dish taste good so you don't have to figure it out by trial and error. Keep these sources handy in the kitchen for when you want to cook healthy meals.

Principle #130

Replace high-fat condiments with low-fat options.

———————————— ✳ ————————————

A lot of people do not consider condiments as "foods" even though they can pack more calories than their main meal. The most common additives that can add significant calories are mayonnaise, sauces, aioli, sour cream, cheese, butter, and salad dressing. A single tablespoon of mayonnaise has 100 calories and 11 grams of fat. A typical recipe for potato salad calls for half a cup of mayonnaise. This condiment alone accounts for 800 calories and 89 grams of fat. If you are not careful about the extras, you may be eating options that may seem healthy but are really sabotaging your weight-loss efforts.

Principle #131

Choose whole fruits rather than juice.

Whole fruits can help you lose weight. Fruits contain essential phytonutrients and their fiber and water content help you feel satisfied. Commercial fruit juice often contains added sugars, so you end up taking in more calories. Also, when the pulp and skin of the fruit is removed, the sugar absorbs quickly within the body and can cause cravings later in the day. Juicing removes the bulk of the fruit so juice does not fill you up like the fruit does. Half of a large grapefruit has 50 calories, 2 grams of fiber, and 11 grams of sugar while 8 fluid ounces of grapefruit juice contains about 100 calories and 22 grams of sugar.

Principle #132

Switch from white to whole grain breads and pasta.

Research has shown that switching from white flour to whole grains is one of the most beneficial changes you can make when losing weight. White flour can increase your appetite and make you gain weight. Whole grains can help you lose weight in the following ways: First, they are digested slowly so they keep your energy levels steady. Second, they contain high amounts of fiber that make you feel full. Studies also show that people who eat three or more servings of whole grains a day have lower body mass indexes and are twice as more likely to maintain their weight over time.

WHAT TO DO WHEN DINING OUT

A recent survey found that 86 percent of dieters said that dining out represented the biggest challenge to their diet. While able to stick to their diet at home, at work, and even at friends' houses, once in a restaurant, their diet quickly unraveled. Why does dining out present such a challenge to so many dieters?

One reason is that restaurant food is cooked primarily with your palate in mind, not your waistline. Indeed, chefs go to great lengths to include sauces, batters, and other calorie-laden accessories to dishes to improve their flavor and presentation.

A second reason dining out on a diet is tricky is because you cannot control the meal's ingredients. For example, if you made yourself a hamburger at home, you might choose a low-fat burger, or maybe even substitute it with a turkey or Veggie burger. You might choose a low-fat or multi-grain bun, skip the cheese, and serve it with a small side salad. But in a restaurant, you will be served a big, dripping, quarter pound, sometimes even a third-of-a-pound, hamburger. The burger could be topped with special sauces, cheese, and bacon and served with potato or pasta salad on the side. Once these items are in front of you, you will surely be tempted to eat them. Therefore, when dining out you must make an extra effort to control the ingredients of the meal you order the same way you would control the ingredients of the meal you make at home.

Luckily, American restaurants are beginning to accommodate the public's newfound interest in losing weight. National chains now offer healthy or low-cal dishes or make other changes that help the calorie-conscious have a pleasant dining experience. For example, Applebee's® menu lists calorie, fat, and fiber content for dishes right on the menu. Similarly, Chili's® offers the "Guiltless Grill®" that features fresh grilled pitas, platters, and sandwiches for around 500 calories a plate. The following simple principles are sure to arm you with the tools you need to have a satisfying yet healthy dining experience.

PRINCIPLE #133

Order your take-out in advance.

Ask restaurants both near your home and work to fax you take-out menus. Check if they post menus on line. Many restaurants now include nutritional information or have a section for healthy diners on their websites. Highlight only the entrees that fit within your diet. If you have to order take-out, make this decision early in the day and call in the order ahead of time. Most restaurants will ask when you want the food to be ready for pick up. Waiting until you are starving will make it hard to stick with your healthy options. Serve a portion of your take-out on a plate and then put the rest of it away.

PRINCIPLE #134

Check the nutrition information for fast food.

If you have a craving for fast food, go to the restaurant's Web site and look up the fat and calorie content before you buy it. The nutritional value of fast food is usually counterproductive for losing weight. However, checking the nutritional content for menu items online can help you make a list of the healthiest options at your typical restaurants. Some of these Web sites also have features where you can track the total nutritional content of a meal you create. Make a list of acceptable foods and the number of calories for your desired meals. You can decide what fits into your diet before you order.

Principle #135

Don't leave home hungry.

---- ✳ ----

Have a small snack before you go out to eat or attend a social event where appetizers and drinks will be served. If you are headed somewhere that serves easily accessible food, it's harder to resist when you are famished. Try to eat something small and healthy so you don't make bad choices or munch all night. Choose a snack with a lot of protein so you feel full longer. This will help keep your hunger in control when faced with a selection of tasty foods. Slices of turkey or chicken, low-fat yogurt, reduced-fat cheese, or a protein smoothie taste great and will keep you satisfied while you lose weight.

PRINCIPLE #136

Order off the menu instead of getting the buffet.

Buffets are tempting because of the value, the selection of foods, and the option to go for seconds. It can be extremely difficult to practice portion control for a single dish, let alone resist the wide array of foods, drinks, and desserts presented at buffets! The standard buffet has over 100 different options. The uncontrolled variety at buffets and the mentality that you can eat as much as you want can derail the most disciplined dieter. Instead of heading to the buffet, take a look at the menu so you can limit what you eat. Most buffets also have a house menu where you can order single items.

PRINCIPLE #137

Share an entrée.

---- ✳ ----

Studies show that the more food you are served, the more you eat. One study showed that participants who consumed larger portions did not report feeling fuller afterward. Restaurants are serving portions so large these days that the practice is being scrutinized by the government. Health institutions claim that one factor contributing to increasing obesity rates is oversized portions. Many restaurants are famous for their huge portions and serve two to three times the amount of food an average person needs. Lose weight by splitting an entree with a friend. Most restaurant portions will satisfy two people. However, keep in mind that many restaurants may charge you extra to split a plate.

PRINCIPLE #138

Put down the menu.

See if the restaurant has an on line menu. Select your meal before your appetite or the smell or sight of food entices you to stray from your diet. Bypass the menu when you arrive at the restaurant. Menus are designed to make dishes sound appealing so patrons order and eat more. Research also shows that taking a look at the dessert menu can double your chances of ordering dessert. Be aware of all the different places food is advertised, such as the separate drink and appetizer menu, daily specials, and place mats. If you start to feel tempted by advertisements, simply ask the server to remove them.

Principle #139

Resist the sales pitch.

Refuse tempting presentations or specials when losing weight. The larger the bill, the more money the restaurant makes. As a result, servers are trained to describe their dishes in the most appealing terms. Many restaurants offer employees bonuses if they sell non-entree items such as dessert, appetizers, and drinks. For example, instead of asking, "What would you like to drink?" they may say, "We have a frozen strawberry margarita that would be perfect with some chips and guacamole." People also have the tendency to be more convinced to order dessert than other items. Tell the sever that you are not interested in looking at the dessert menu or not to bring the dessert tray.

PRINCIPLE #140

Know how a dish is prepared.

※

A seemingly harmless meal can be loaded with hidden fat and calories unless you know exactly how it is prepared. Look out for high-calorie preparation methods such as breading, deep frying, or pan frying. Choose fish or chicken prepared in the following ways to lose weight: steamed, poached, roasted, broiled, boiled, grilled, or baked. Skip the sauce or glaze. Honey and maple glazes are often full of sugar while cream-based sauces are high in fat. Most meals come with vegetables. Ask if they are sautéed in butter. If they are, order your vegetables steamed instead. If you have any doubts on how a dish is prepared ask your server.

PRINCIPLE #141

Entertain with healthy options.

Create a menu that includes healthy, lower-calorie options rather than serving standard party foods. Some healthy hors d'oeuvres include shrimp cocktail, chicken skewers, crudités with low-fat dip, baked or sweet potato chips, a fruit tray, and sparkling water. Prepare dips with fat-free yogurt or sour cream. For picnics and barbecues, choose lean cuts of meat that have less fat, such as flank steak, or trim off excess fat before cooking. Instead of ground beef burgers, use ground turkey. Offer a few healthy dessert options, such as a parfait with low-fat granola and berries with light whip cream for those who want to lose weight.

Principle #142

Ask for the soup of the day.

Research has indicated that eating broth-based soup with fiber like vegetable soup before your main entree can result in eating less of your main course. A study was completed where participants ate a 250 calorie first course before eating their lunch. The participants were separated into three groups. The first group had a casserole. The second group had a casserole plus 10 ounces of water to drink. And the third group was served a soup containing 10 ounces of water. The results showed that the soup-eating group ate about 100 fewer calories at lunch. This group did not feel hungrier and they did not eat additional calories later to compensate for the lower-calorie meal.

Principle #143

Order shrimp cocktail as an appetizer.

One of the most healthful appetizers that you can order and still lose weight is shrimp cocktail. Most appetizers are deep fried and full of fat. Resist eating deep-fried appetizers. A 3 ounce serving of fresh shrimp has 84 calories, 17 grams of protein, and less than a gram of fat. But if you order shrimp breaded and deep fried, you end up with 206 calories and 10 grams of fat. Even though cocktail sauce has less fat than many other dips, it can still contain added sugar. Squeeze a fresh lemon over shrimp instead to enhance the flavor. The high protein content of shrimp will help you feel full longer.

Principle #144

Be smart when ordering a salad.

———— ✳ ————

It is important to note that when dining out, salads aren't always the answer. In fact, some salads have more fat, calories, and sodium than other menu items. In some restaurants, a Cobb Salad (made with egg, bacon, and cheese) with ranch dressing contains 950 calories and 25 grams of fat. In addition, many salads are topped with bacon bits and croutons, which further add calories, fat, and sodium. If you do order a salad, choose one that is topped with a low-fat meat (such as grilled chicken or salmon). Always order dressing on the side, and then use it sparingly.

Principle #145

Eat to lose weight even during special gatherings.

Be aware of your diet during special occasions. The following are some suggestions to help you get through social situations where food is involved. Place yourself the farthest away from serving tables and trays. Be social and engage in conversation with family and friends. Step away from the dinner table when you are done eating or have the server clear your plate. Keep mints handy to prevent nibbling on food. Alternate a drink with a glass of sparking water and lime to prevent excess calories from alcohol.

PRINCIPLE #146

Ask your server to remove the bread basket.

The bread served at restaurants is one of the leading causes of overeating. The average amount of bread and butter eaten with dinner can add up to 500 calories to your meal. To lose weight and prevent mindlessly picking at these items, have the server take bread away. Or if you really can't resist, take a single serving and place it on you side plate before removing the basket. Use olive oil rather than butter for bread. Studies have shown that diners who eat bread with olive oil end up eating fewer calories from this combination than those who butter their bread.

PRINCIPLE #147

Order authentic Mexican food.

You can still enjoy this delicious cuisine and lose weight if you know the ways you can cut fat and calories. Bypass the basket of tortilla chips. A regular restaurant basket can contain up to 700 calories and 33 grams of fat. Leave the salsa to use on your main dish. With only 25 calories per 4 ounce serving, salsa is a great replacement for other high-fat condiments and sauces such as guacamole and sour cream. Have the grilled chicken or fish soft tacos instead of beef. Skip white or creamy sauces that are high in fat. Order corn rather than flour tortillas and black beans rather than refried beans.

Principle #148

Be choosy with Chinese foods.

———————————— ✳ ————————————

Choose steamed appetizers such as dim sum or dumplings over anything fried. If you like fried wontons, wonton soup is a wise alternative. Anything batter dipped, deep fried, and covered in a sugary sauce is automatically off limits as a main course. These dishes include General Taos's chicken, orange, mandarin, sweet and sour beef or chicken. A combination meal of fried rice, noodles, spring roll, and one of the items above contains around 900 calories and 40 grams of fat. A better choice to lose weight would be a stir-fry meal with steamed rice, Chinese vegetables, and chicken with black bean sauce at 550 calories and 13 grams of fat.

PRINCIPLE #149

Resist the temptations when ordering Italian foods.

You can enjoy the ambiance of your favorite Italian restaurant and still lose weight if you skip the bread basket. Healthy appetizers include shrimp cocktail or grilled calamari. Italian soups such as minestrone are filled with vegetables and fiber and can be extremely satisfying. Choose a garden salad over a Caesar, which has 520 calories and 43 grams of fat. If you order pasta, see if they have a whole-wheat option and ask for a half portion. Tomato sauce contains the antioxidant lycopene and is lower in fat and calories than cream based sauce. Avoid pesto, parmigiana, alfredo and baked pasta dishes, as these contain high amounts of cheese, butter, and fat.

PRINCIPLE #150

Order the basics when eating "All-American food."

If you take away all the bells and whistles that have been added to American cuisine, you will find that the basic ingredients are actually quite healthy. Start off by selecting moderate portions. For meat and potatoes, take away all the extras and you end up with a well rounded, low calorie meal. Select lean cuts of beef like "round" or "loin" as in round roast or sirloin. The standard serving size for meat is 3 ounces. Most restaurants serve 8 to 14 ounce portions. Choose the smallest option and only eat half. Round out your meal with a plain baked potato and steamed broccoli at only 350 calories and 5 grams of fat.

PRINCIPLE #151

Take half of your food to go.

If you only eat half of the food that you order in restaurants, you automatically cut in half your potential total caloric intake. Ask the server to split the meal and wrap half in advance. When your food is already tucked away, you are less likely to pick at leftover food when you have finished eating. You can plan on having the leftovers for dinner or save them for a quick lunch the following day. Requesting half your meal to go means that you've already planned for your next meal. This is one less food decision that you have to make to lose weight.

Principle #152

You don't have to clean your plate.

Polls have indicated that over 50 percent of Americans make a habit of cleaning their plate. People tend to eat whatever is placed in front of them. For many people, habit forces them to continue eating even though they are already full. If you're like most people who have made a habit of cleaning their plate, try eating off of smaller plates to lose weight. One serving of pasta equals 1/2 cup of cooked pasta. However, most restaurants serve a pasta dish with up to 4 servings. You do not need to clean off the plate every time. You can simply ask to take home the leftovers.

PRINCIPLE #153

Ask for healthy modifications.

———————————— ✳ ————————————

Just because the menu says that a dish is fried doesn't mean you have to order it that way. Most restaurants are more than willing to accommodate special requests. There are many adjustments that you can make to high-calorie restaurant foods to make them work with your diet. Order deep fried or pan fried meats grilled, baked, or broiled instead. For dishes that come with cream-based sauce, ask if they have an alternative like a mango salsa. For dishes that are "au gratin," have them replace the cheese sauce with a little bit of grated Parmesan. Most entrees come with two sides. Save some calories by requesting a double portion of steamed veggies instead of rice or potatoes.

Principle #154

Be prepared to send your food back.

---　✳　---

Eating to lose weight at restaurants involves knowing what to ask for and then making sure you get it. If you have ordered something not on the menu or have asked for modifications or substitutions, communicate clearly so that the server understands exactly what you want. He or she will be able to make sure the kitchen follows through with your order. Since restaurants are used to preparing meals based on menu descriptions, your modifications may be overlooked. Don't feel like you need to eat something that you did not ask for. Speak up, be polite, and request that your meal be sent back and prepared the way you ordered it.

Principle #155

Drink water or unsweetened tea.

Restaurants rack up the bill not only through food but also through high-priced specialty drinks and beverages. A regular 16 ounce soft drink contains almost 200 calories. With free refills throughout the meal, you can easily drink over 600 calories worth of soda. In addition to excess calories, alcohol may weaken your determination to stick to your diet. Alcohol is also processed for energy first, followed by carbohydrates, protein, then fat. Consuming large amounts of alcohol with a high-fat meal means that the excess calories can get stored as fat. Stick with water with your meal to lose weight, or have a glass of unsweetened ice tea with lemon.

PRINCIPLE #156

Ask for dressing on the side.

---- ✳ ----

Condiments, sauces, and dressings are often high in calories. These sauces contain large amounts of butter, cream, fat, and sugar. Restaurants also pour these liberally on salads, appetizers, and entrees. The standard serving size for dressing and sauces is 2 tablespoons, around 150 calories and 15 grams of fat. The average restaurant pours on 4 or more tablespoons at 350 calories and 37 grams of fat. Instead of cream dressings like Caesar, blue cheese, and ranch, ask for a light or fat-free version or vinaigrette on the side to cut calories and lose weight. Dip your fork in the dressing before spearing your salad to add a little flavor.

PRINCIPLE #157

Order fruit for dessert.

———————— ✳ ————————

Refined sugar and flour, butter, fat, cream, and oils found in desserts should all be avoided when you want to lose weight. For example, a molten chocolate cake with vanilla ice cream has an astounding 1,270 calories and 62 grams of fat A popular chain serves a carrot cake with over 1,500 calories and 84 grams of fat per slice. Ask your server how many calories are in the dessert that you are thinking about ordering. Once you know how many calories it has, it may be easier to pass it up. Ask if they offer a better option. While fresh fruit may not even be on the menu, ask the server if they can bring out a plate of whatever fruits they have in season.

ADOPTING HABITS
OF SLIM PEOPLE

Do you have a friend who always passes on dessert, while you count down the minutes to treating yourself to a cookie or ice cream at the end of the day? What about someone in your family who loses 10 pounds without even trying, while you struggle with all your might just to lose a couple pounds? It seems that all of us know at least someone who has an easy time losing weight, or even more infuriating, someone who is so slim he or she has never even had to think about it at all! Part of this person's easy relationship with their weight can be attributed to genes. Indeed, some of us simply inherit high metabolic rates or extremely muscular body types, which offer natural weight-loss advantages.

Yet naturally slender people also tend to have different lifestyles than do those who need to actively try to lose weight. They are less likely to use food as an emotional crutch or to resort to eating when bored, nervous, or impatient. They are also more likely to be naturally drawn to physical activities that keep their metabolism high and their muscles working. Most important, they tend to think differently about hunger, and thus make different choices when considering what foods to eat, when to eat them, and how much of them to eat.

It makes good sense, then, to mimic the habits of slim people. What works for them can also work for you as you continue to change your habits and lifestyle to achieve a thinner you. The following principles will help you learn to think and act like a slender person, putting you on the fast track toward weight loss.

PRINCIPLE #158

Keep a food journal.

— ✳ —

Keeping track of what you eat and drink, monitoring your food decisions, emotions, and hunger levels, is crucial to your weight loss success. A food diary is a comprehensive daily reminder weight loss plan. Your daily journal can help you stay focused on your personal goals and keep you motivated toward your weight loss target. You will be able to keep track of your food and beverage intake, make sure you are within your daily calorie allotment, and ensure that you are getting enough fluids. You should also log your physical fitness activities, supplements, energy levels and daily weight. This ongoing routine will make it easier to lose weight. The best journal on the market is titled *I Will Lose Weight This Time Diet Journal* by Alex Lluch.

Principle #159

Choose being satisfied over being stuffed.

Most people who are able to maintain their weight finish eating when they feel neither hungry nor full. Those who are overweight tend to continue eating past the point of comfort. The next time you eat, periodically stop and put down your utensils. Notice how your stomach feels. Can you stop eating now and feel satisfied? Find out if it is true hunger or habit that is driving you to finish your meal. If you are used to eating past the point of comfort, gradually cut back on portions and eat more slowly until you get used to stopping at a comfortable level.

Principle #160

Don't view hunger as good or bad.

Hunger is just your body's natural signal to fuel itself. People tend to read into their hunger more than they need to. Thin people look at hunger as a simple signal from their bodies that they need food for energy. Most people who carry extra weight view hunger as a condition to be avoided. Therefore, overweight people consistently overeat or eat even when they don't have any natural signals to do so. Thin people recognize their hunger and understand where these sensations are coming from. If you find yourself eating for no reason, try skipping a snack. You may realize that you didn't even need it.

Principle #161

Satisfy emotional needs through methods other than food.

The five typical emotions or states that cause overeating are loneliness, boredom, anger, stress, and fatigue. Those who are thin are able to catch themselves when eating out of emotion and stop before they overeat. If your are truly hungry, have a 100-200 calorie snack like a teaspoon of peanut butter on whole wheat toast. You should feel an immediate boost in your energy. Find non-food related ways to satisfy emotional needs. Stay connected with friends and family who know you are trying to lose weight. Exercise to relieve stress and don't stay up too late at night.

Principle #162

Eat more fruit.

A study based on the nutritional habits of lean people showed that they have an additional serving of fruit, consume more fiber, and have less fat per day than people who are overweight. The additional serving of fruit may account for the difference in weight since fruit naturally is low-fat and high in fiber. It's bulk and sweetness may satisfy lean people with a lot less calories than cookies and pastries consumed by heavier individuals. Include two to three servings of fruit each day. Keep easy-to-eat fruits such as apples, oranges, and bananas in visible places in your kitchen and office so they are handy for when you need a snack.

Principle #163

Know what foods you can eat safely and stick to them.

Predictability and routine are key aspects of the eating patterns of lean people. Those who manage their weight tend to be consistent in the types of food they eat. Create a routine that revolves around the same type of food for each of your major meals and snacks. These decisions will eventually become second nature. For example, to lose weight, loosely plan on having cereal for breakfast, a sandwich at lunch, and a salad for dinner. Keep meals from being monotonous by changing the ingredients for each meal.

Principle #164

Practice self-control.

One of the most significant behavioral indicators of weight gain is a lack of self-control. Studies show that people who had honed their self-restraint had the lowest body mass index. On the other hand, a low level of restraint has been linked to weight gain of up to 30 pounds in adults. Learn to control your appetite. Plan ahead for situations where you have traditionally lacked self-control, such as parties and social events. Decide in advance what you will and will not eat. Pass on alcohol since it lowers inhibitions.

Principle #165

Stay active.

Studies show that on average, slim people move around 2 ½ more hours a week than those who are overweight. This extra activity can account for an additional weight loss of 2-3 pounds a month. Figure out exactly how much you move around a day. If you have an office job where the majority of your day is spent at a desk, you can end up spending most of your day sitting. You sit while driving, at work, during meals, and while watching TV. Balance out this inactivity by walking around more. Your daily activities should involve taking 10,000 steps a day. Wear a pedometer to see how your steps add up.

Principle #166

Get extra sleep.

People who have less body fat get around two more hours of sleep a week versus those who carry more weight. Researchers suggest that increased body weight from lack of sleep is linked to our hormones. As mentioned before, sleep deprivation decreases the amounts of leptin in our system. Leptin is a hormone that suppresses hunger. If we don't get enough sleep, the body increases the levels of ghrelin, an appetite-boosting hormone. Make sure your hormones are at the proper levels for weight loss. Try going to bed 17 minutes earlier than your typical bedtime. Eventually you want to aim for eight hours of sleep on most nights of the week to lose weight.

PRINCIPLE #167

Stick with your diet on the weekends.

※

People who maintain their weight eat consistently seven days of the week. Follow your diet throughout the week, especially on weekends, to lose weight at a steady pace. One study found that individuals who weigh more eat more on the weekends than they do during the week. Participants showed that these individuals consumed over 100 more calories each day on Friday, Saturday, and Sunday than they did Monday through Thursday. Maintaining the same eating patterns for all days of the week will help you establish these choices as long-term habits.

FOODS AND SUPPLEMENTS THAT HELP YOU LOSE WEIGHT

An old wives' tale says that if you break all of your food in half, the calories will fall out. Of course, breaking your candy bar in half will never cause it to lose the hundreds of calories it contains. As we said before, certain kinds of foods like celery, lettuce, and cabbage contain so few calories that your body burns more calories chewing and digesting them. Such foods are referred to as "negatively caloric" and can be great for keeping your mouth busy and your body trim.

Still other foods are processed so efficiently by the body that they too facilitate weight loss. Protein, for example, keeps you full and increases your energy, which leads to overall weight loss. Protein also helps build muscle, which is the body's calorie-burning factory. Indeed, the more muscle you have, the more quickly and efficiently you will burn calories and lose weight. Consider that a pound of muscle burns about 6 calories a day, while a pound of fat burns only 2 calories a day. Therefore, a person made up of more muscle than fat will burn three times more calories doing the same activities, because his muscular body is working more efficiently.

Similarly, foods rich in fiber should be eaten because they help aid weight loss. Fiber is the part of plant-based foods that our bodies are unable to digest. Fiber passes through our digestive tract without providing nutrition or calories, so this roughage does a lot of beneficial work for little "cost." Fiber helps the body eliminate waste, which keeps your systems clean and clear. When your colon and intestines are clear, your body is able to absorb more of your food's nutrients and more efficiently eliminate toxins.

The following principles identify foods and supplements that help you lose weight. Familiarize yourself with them so you can use them as your ally as you work toward your weight loss goals.

Principle #168

Have protein with every meal.

✳

Eat more protein to help you lose weight. Protein keeps you feeling full, gives you a steady release of energy, and helps build lean muscle tissue. These three factors will help you control your appetite and drop pounds. Good news for those over 40 years of age: additional protein can also result in lower abdominal fat. Opt for lean sources of protein such as chicken, turkey, fish, and shrimp. Other non-animal sources of protein are beans, lentils, chickpeas, low-fat yogurt, and fat-free milk. Nuts are a good source of protein but are high in fat. Limit peanuts and almonds to 1-ounce servings. Be sure to balance your protein intake with other nutrients.

Principle #169

Take a multivitamin.

— ❋ —

Busy schedules make it challenging to get the proper nutrients while losing weight. Because you will be eating less, make up for any areas that are nutritionally deficient by taking a daily multivitamin. A high quality supplement with vitamin C should take care of all your basic requirements. Take your vitamin first thing in the morning with breakfast. You are more likely to forget if you wait until later in the day. Ask your primary care physician or dietitian about the types of supplements you should be taking while on your diet. He or she will be able to tell you exactly what vitamins and minerals you need.

Principle #170

Eat an apple a day to lose weight.

Apples are a simple, convenient, and inexpensive food that you should include in your weight loss plan. Apples contain a substance called pectin that helps you feel satisfied. Pectin is a soluble fiber that provides bulk and is slow to digest. So even though apples contain sugar, the fiber in apples allows the sugar to be released into the bloodstream at a steady rate. Studies show that 5 grams of pectin is enough to leave people feeling full for up to four hours. Eat two apples a day to provide lasting fullness for around 160 calories.

Principle #171

Fortify your body with calcium.

Calcium can increase the rate at which you lose weight. Three to four servings of low-fat dairy a day has been linked to reduced body fat. Though calcium supplements have also been shown to aid weight loss, the calcium from low-fat dairy produced higher levels of fat burning. If you cannot tolerate milk products, try other food sources of calcium, such as dark, leafy greens, salmon, almonds, or oatmeal. Calcium supplements should be combined with vitamin D, zinc, and magnesium, which helps increase the absorption rate. Aim for 1,000–1,300 mg of calcium daily to burn more fat.

Principle #172

Add black beans to your diet.

— ❋ —

Black beans are an excellent source of both protein and complex carbohydrates, which are two essential components of a weight loss meal plan. They are also low in fat and high in nutrients such as fiber and iron. In addition to lowering cholesterol, the high fiber content in black beans make them a "slow burning" food. They digest at a steady rate. This prevents blood sugar levels from spiking after a meal. Black beans are also rich in antioxidants, folate, and magnesium, which are nutrients essential for good health. A cup of black beans has 180 calories, less than a gram of fat, and about 12 grams of fiber and 14 grams of protein.

Principle #173

Replace fatty meats with fish.

Switching from beef to fish can help you lose weight. Fish is full of protein and healthy oils such as omega-3 and is low in calories. Unlike saturated fats that are bad for your heart and your weight, omega-3 may aid in weight loss. Studies show that eating fish may also increase the body's sensitivity to leptin, the hormone that triggers the body to suppress the appetite and burn fat. Fish has been found to keep your blood sugar and insulin levels steady. A 3 ounce serving of cooked halibut has 119 calories and 2.5 grams of fat, while ground beef has 210 calories and 14 grams of fat.

PRINCIPLE #174

Curb cravings with peanut butter.

While nuts are high in calories, researchers theorize that a moderate amount of the healthy fat in nuts may promote satiety. Curbing hunger is important for managing weight loss. Peanut butter keeps you feeling full for hours at a time. You are less likely to overeat later in the day if you have a serving of peanut butter in the morning. According to one study, those who ate peanuts had a lower body mass index than those who refrained from eating nuts. Nuts have healthy fats, vitamins, and minerals, and each serving provides 8 grams of protein for energy while losing weight.

PRINCIPLE #175

Try adding soy as a source of protein.

Soy is an extremely versatile food that can help you lose weight. Soy is a good substitute for many foods because it delivers high quality protein, B-vitamins and iron, and other nutrients for a fraction of the fat and calories. Have your breakfast cereal with unsweetened soy milk instead of whole milk and save 65 calories. Snack on soy crisps with your lunch instead of potato chips and save 40 calories. Make a burger with a soy patty rather than beef and save 110 calories. You can also replace high fat ingredients such as cream sauces with soy or use soy as a substitute in cheesy casseroles and side dishes.

PRINCIPLE #176

Add healthy fats in moderation.

------------------------------------- ❋ -------------------------------------

Dietary fat is required to maintain good health. However, Americans typically eat the wrong types of fat. Research shows that good, monounsaturated fats and omega-3 fatty acids help you lose weight. These fats help build body tissue and cells and allow your body to absorb nutrients. Studies show that omega-3 fats help control the appetite and increase the number of calories burned from fat. Some healthy sources of monounsaturated fats are olive oil, peanuts, cashews, hazelnuts, macadamia nuts, and pine nuts. You can find omega-3s in fatty fish such as salmon, in flaxseed, and in dark leafy greens like kale and collard greens.

Principle #177

Eat orange-colored
fruits and vegetables.

Bright orange fruits and vegetables such as sweet potatoes can aid your efforts to lose weight. Sweet potatoes contain carotenoids that may help stabilize blood sugar levels, lower insulin resistance, and reduce cravings. These foods have high amounts of fiber, which makes you feel satisfied for longer periods of time. Some researchers suggest that the vitamins in these fruits and vegetables help reduce abdominal fat. Antioxidants, such as vitamin C and beta-carotene, may play a role in keeping your belly trim. Carrots, cantaloupe, squash, and peaches are great sources of beta-carotene while oranges are a great source of vitamin C.

Principle #178

Have eggs for breakfast.

--- ✳ ---

Studies show that having eggs in the morning may help you lose up to two pounds a month. Research indicates that eggs help you feel satisfied longer so you end up eating less food the rest of the day. Participants who ate two scrambled eggs with toast and low-calorie fruit spread consumed fewer calories for lunch and dinner compared to participants who had a bagel containing the same amount of calories as the egg breakfast. Studies also show that the protein in eggs may keep your blood sugar and appetite steady. One large egg provides zinc, iron, and vitamins A, D, E, and B12, and contains 78 calories.

CREATING THE RIGHT ENVIRONMENT

We tend to overlook the impact our environment has on us when trying to lose weight. But our surroundings affect our mood, thoughts, and activities, for better or worse. Creating an environment that facilitates weight loss is therefore a key ingredient to achieving your weight-loss goals.

Think of your environment as another tool in your weight-loss arsenal. Some of the tools you have at your disposal are your ability to plan meals, your gym membership, and the weight-loss behaviors and habits you adopt. But the positive impact of each of these tools can be instantly nullified when you put yourself in an environment that makes weight loss more difficult. If your home or office is filled with fatty snacks, your diet will become derailed. If you surround yourself with overeating stimuli, such as large dishes, television, fast-paced music and even bright lights and colors (which studies show increases the pace at which we consume food), no matter how much time you spent on the treadmill that morning, you will end up overeating or eating poorly that night.

Your home or office can be made weight-loss friendly in just a few hours. At home, remove all junk food from the fridge and pantry, replacing chips and cookies with healthy snacks such as carrot sticks or nuts. Keep portions of healthy foods frozen so they are ready to go. Keep the same healthy snacks you stock in your home kitchen at your office. Indeed, many of us blow our diet during the last few hours of work, when hunger overtakes us. Remove all of your change from your drawers so you are unable to hit up the vending machine for salty chips or chocolate bars. Replace it with dried fruits or microwave popcorn, which is excellent for satisfying daytime snacking urges. Above all, avoid letting your environment undermine your attempts to lose weight. Use these and the principles that follow to create surroundings that help you lose weight.

Principle #179

Clear your kitchen of junk foods.

Remove junk foods from your cupboards, refrigerator, and freezer. When favorite foods are easily accessible, you will be constantly fighting temptation. Junk foods have very little nutritional value, are high in calories, and include artificial flavors and preservatives. Junk foods also contain ingredients that are bad for weight loss such as trans fats, high-fructose corn syrup, and refined carbohydrates. Go through your kitchen and remove foods like candy, sugary cereals, high-fat potato and corn chips, soda, packaged cookies, pastries, and desserts. Restock your kitchen with healthier, low-calorie options such as low-fat popcorn, apples, whole-wheat crackers and high-fiber cereals that will help you lose weight.

PRINCIPLE #180

Keep food out of sight.

Research suggests that looking at tempting food can increase the chances that you will eat it. Seeing a food that you enjoy can actually trigger a pleasure chemical in the brain called dopamine. Dopamine is associated with feelings of pleasure and reward. Just the sight of food causes a significant increase in levels of this neurotransmitter and increases our desire to eat the food we look at. Place high-calorie foods such as candy in opaque rather than clear containers. Better yet, remove them from your immediate vicinity. One study showed that the consumption of candy decreased from nine pieces to four pieces as the candy was placed farther away.

Principle #181

Stock your pantry
with ingredients not snacks.

Encourage yourself to cook healthy meals by keeping ingredients such as olive oil, beans, bags of grains, herbs, spices, and canned vegetables in the cupboards that are the most convenient to reach. In most pantries, the worst foods are often the most accessible foods. Don't place easy-to-eat snacks in plain sight or in cupboards that you frequently open. Store snacks in a secondary cabinet that you access on rare occasions. Stock up on ingredients for healthy meals such as: black, kidney, and pinto beans; chickpeas and lentils; brown and wild rice; canned items, such as tuna, vegetables, soups; nuts and nut butters.

Principle #182

Turn off the music.

───────── ✳ ─────────

Different types of music may cause you to consume more calories than if you eat in silence. One study showed that participants who ate with music playing in the background spent ten more minutes eating and ended up consuming 450 additional calories versus participants who ate without music. The speed of music can also affect the rate at which you eat. Upbeat music can make you eat faster so you end up eating more food in less time. Relaxing music makes you chew more thoroughly and spend more time tasting your food. However, you can still end up eating more because soft music encourages longer mealtimes. Turn the music off and have a conversation instead.

PRINCIPLE #183

Adjust the lighting.

———————————— ✳ ————————————

Bright lights can increase your stress levels and encourage you to eat faster than normal. Research shows that bright light, such as the florescent bulbs typically used in fast food restaurants, can cause you to eat faster. If you have to eat in a brightly lit restaurant, remind yourself to eat slowly. Control your atmosphere at home so your dining area is neither too bright, nor too dark. A darker room decreases your self-restraint and leaves you more susceptible to temptation. Low lighting also reduces your ability to pay attention to what you're eating. Change your dining atmosphere so it's conducive to weight loss. Switch your light bulbs to 60-75 watt incandescent bulbs.

Principle #184

Keep your dining room neutral.

Paint your dining room walls in beige, white, and grays to prevent overeating. Restaurants use color theory to encourage diners to eat quickly and leave or to encourage diners to linger over their meal and eat more. Studies show that intense reds, oranges, and yellows can increase feelings of hunger and thirst. These colors make your dining area more stimulating so you'll want to eat quickly. Cool colors such as blues and greens encourage you to spend more time on your food. Additional time at the table opens up the possibility of eating more foods. Stick with basic, neutral colors in your dining room to lose weight.

PRINCIPLE #185

Spend a half an hour for mealtimes.

Spend too little or too much time on your meals and you may end up eating more than you need. Your brain needs around 20 minutes to recognize that your stomach is full. If you eat too quickly, your brain will not receive the signals to stop eating. If you eat your lunch in less than ten minutes, you may reach for more food before you recognize that you're full. Also, don't linger around food after you've had enough. Spending more than 20-30 minutes on your meals means that you are likely to pick at your leftovers. Take a half an hour on your meals so you can enjoy your food, but not be tempted for more.

Principle #186

Turn off the TV.

---------- ✳ ----------

Over 90 percent of Americans watch TV while dining at home. People who watch television while eating tend to overeat without being aware of it. Studies have shown that people can eat almost an entire extra meal's worth of calories on days where they ate in front of the TV. Television distracts eaters from responding naturally to their body's cues of hunger and fullness. Turning on the TV can trigger you to want a snack even if you are not hungry. You also tend to rely on external cues, such as the end of a show, rather than internal cues to stop eating. Keep the TV off and sit down at the table to savor the flavor, color, and texture of your food.

Principle #187

Distract your nose.

--- ✳ ---

There is a reason why pastry shops blow the smell of fresh baked goods onto the sidewalk. Smell enhances our tasting experience and can trigger feelings of hunger. Studies indicate that good-smelling foods can increase consumption. Scent is one of the ways our bodies can tell that food is available. Once we realize that food is nearby, our bodies secrete hormones that make us want to eat. Foods that smell good may make our meal seem to taste better. This appeal may lead to eat more than you need, regardless of your hunger level. A menthol lozenge or lip balm may distract against a tempting smell.

PRINCIPLE #188

Turn off the air conditioning.

—— ❋ ——

People tend to eat more when the temperature is cooler. When you are cold, you attempt to control your body temperature by eating. Your body requires more energy to stabilize its core temperature. The energy comes in the form of food. When people are hot, they sweat to cool down their body temperature. This regulatory process burns calories. Also, people tend to eat less when they are warm. Controlling the temperature of your surroundings through air conditioning means that your body's natural regulatory systems don't have to work. Try raising the temperature of the room to help you eat less and lose weight.

PRINCIPLE #189

Have dinner alone.

— ❋ —

People tend to eat less when dining alone. An individual can consume over 40 percent more food when eating with another person. When dining with others, you can be tempted to stray from your usual choices. The soup and salad you would have normally chosen to eat to lose weight all of a sudden doesn't look as appetizing compared to the fried appetizers your friend ordered. You also have to spend more effort resisting a bite from your friend's plate, especially if he or she insists. Spend your energy focused on your own food without distractions. You will be less likely to be tempted by the choices of others.

EXERCISING TO LOSE WEIGHT

Philosopher Robert M. Hutchins once said, "Whenever I feel like exercising, I lie down until the feeling passes." Hutchins was remarking on something common to many Americans: a dislike for exercise. Indeed, some of us will do anything to avoid exercise. Humorists often joke that if it weren't for the distance between the television and the refrigerator, many of us would get no exercise at all.

Many Americans mistakenly believe that exercise is difficult and unpleasant. Quite the contrary, exercising can be fun and enjoyable. If you hate running on the treadmill at the gym, consider playing a sport such as tennis, baseball, or soccer.

Another misconception Americans often have is that they are too busy to exercise. However, there is always time to exercise if you build it into your daily routine. Try cutting your lunch break in half and go for a brisk walk after your meal. Or, take a walk around your neighborhood before or after dinner. Finally, get exercise through the activities already on your to-do list. In fact, everyday chores, if done properly, can substitute for a more formal exercise routine. For example, an hour of gardening burns approximately 281 calories; vacuuming burns about 246. Get the most out of activities you have to do anyway by incorporating exercise into them. Do squats as you fold laundry. Do arm curls with books as you replace them on shelves around your house. Be on the lookout for ways to turn ordinary chores into exercises that count.

Finally, realize that exercising always makes you feel better. Studies have shown that engaging in frequent exercise will improve your mood in as little as 2 weeks. When you exercise, your body releases endorphins, which naturally elevates your mood and gives you more energy. Your body will become addicted to the natural high that endorphins provide.

The following principles will encourage you to spend more time being active. The better you look and feel, the more exercise you will want to do, further helping your weight loss goals.

Principle #190

Burn calories through exercise.

— ✳ —

Exercise helps you lose weight by increasing the amount of calories you burn. A pound of fat is the equivalent of 3,500 stored calories. To lose weight you have to burn more calories through exercise than you consume. Exercise helps prevent weight gain and facilitates weight loss by burning calories. If you burn 500 more calories daily than you eat, you will lose around a pound a week. Schedule exercise into your daily routine. Incorporate activities such as walking, jogging, or biking into your workouts. Try to include a combination of cardiovascular, strength, and flexibility training 3 to 4 times a week.

Principle #191

Participate in
aerobic activities.

❋

You can double your rate of weight loss by eating a sensible diet and adding regular aerobic activities to your daily routine. One of the main reasons to exercise for weight loss is to burn extra calories. Aerobic exercise improves your physical fitness by increasing the strength of your heart and lungs. It also helps you burn fat. You can lose weight faster if you include activities such as running, dancing, swimming, or kickboxing on a daily basis. The longer and harder you work out, the more calories you burn. One of the most effective ways to lose body fat is to include at least 30 minutes of aerobic exercise five times a week.

Principle #192

Get your mind off the discomfort of exercise.

A little exercise can go a long way to help you lose weight. However, people often stop due to discomfort. When you are tempted to quit, relate the strenuous nature of exercise to weight loss. Breathing, sweating, and an increased heart rate are all by-products of exercise. Take pleasure at challenging yourself. Expect to feel some discomfort and recognize that these sensations are temporary. Focus on the long-term advantages of weight loss. Keep your mind on the aspects of exercise you like. Feel a sense of accomplishment. Enjoy the social interactions that may accompany your routine or enjoy the feeling of being outdoors.

Principle #193

Remember that all weights are not equal.

———————— ✳ ————————

Determine your body composition to find out how much weight you need to lose. You may be thin but have a disproportionate amount of fat. Conversely, you may be losing fat, but your body weight may stay the same due to increased muscle mass. Muscle weighs more than fat, so don't be discouraged if the number on the scale does not change. One of the best ways to lose fat and increase muscle is to build a regular exercise routine into your schedule. Dieting without exercise encourages your body to burn muscle for energy rather than fat. To maximize your weight loss, lose the fat and increase your muscle mass.

PRINCIPLE #194

Vary your exercise routine.

———————————— ✳ ————————————

The body quickly adapts to any activity performed on a regular basis. When you find that your workout routine does not provide the same results as when you first started, it may be that your body has adapted to it. Challenge your body by switching up your routine. Try alternating 20 minutes each on the elliptical machine, stationery bike, and stair climber rather than always using the treadmill. Changing machines requires muscles to exert in different ways, forcing your body to meet the new demand. If you use machines for strength training, switch to free weights. You will use extra energy to stabilize the weights and maintain proper form.

Principle #195

Incorporate "interval training" in your workout routine to maximize weight loss.

Interval training can help boost your resting metabolism and increase your fat-burning potential more than traditional endurance workouts. Interval training alternates short bouts of vigorous activity with a brief recovery period. Interval training pushes your system into anaerobic mode, making it more efficient at utilizing oxygen. The more oxygen you use, the more calories you burn. Interval training strengthens the cardiovascular system and improves endurance. Start by alternating 1-minute sprints with a 3-minute walk. Aim for a 20-30 minute session 2-3 times a week.

Principle #196

Perform high intensity exercises to
continue burning calories
even after you workout.

Studies show that exercises that increase your heart rate over 75 percent of your maximum capacity enable you to burn more calories post exercise. High intensity cardio or heavy weight lifting raises your heart rate and creates an effect scientist refer to as excess post exercise oxygen consumption (EPEOC), commonly knon as "afterburn." Try a 60-minute session at 75-80 p7ercent of your maximum heart rate. Research has indicated that physically fit people who participated in high-intensity exercise burned more calories for several hours after they trained. They also burned almost twice as many calories from fat.

Principle #197

Build muscle to boost your metabolism.

In addition to strengthening and building muscle, weight training can also help you burn more calories by increasing your resting metabolism. Your resting metabolic rate is the rate at which you burn calories to maintain the basic functions of your body. Muscle tissue burns the most calories. If you add muscle, your body will burn around 50 more calories for every pound of muscle you gain. You can lose weight quicker and more easily by increasing your lean muscle mass than through dieting alone. Studies have shown that consistent weight training can boost your metabolic rate by almost 15 percent. Lift weights for 20 minutes 3 times a week to see results.

Principle #198

Work out first thing
in the morning.

Wake up early to exercise, and you will be less likely to skip your workout after a long day. Studies show that working out first thing in the morning can help you burn more calories from fat. When you are sleeping, your body is in fasting mode. Upon waking up, your body's energy reserves are depleted. Exercising in the morning makes your body burn fat for energy. Cardio in the morning can elevate your metabolism for several hours after the workout is over. Exercising also improves your mood and increases your alertness. Working out may also help regulate your eating patterns and prevent overeating the rest of the day.

PRINCIPLE #199

Fuel your workout with the proper foods.

Eat the right foods to ensure you have enough energy to workout. There is no sense in working out if your body can't keep up. The key is to eat foods that fuel your workout and enable you to lose weight at the same time. Have a small protein-filled snack several hours before a cardio workout to ensure you have the energy to last through the whole routine. Protein takes longer to digest so your body will need to rely on stored fat in addition to food for energy. Keep snacks between 100 to 200 calories. A perfect snack is two slices of turkey on half a slice of whole wheat bread with lettuce and mustard.

Principle #200

Keep up with your routine.

Exercise is a crucial aspect of weight loss. Don't rely on your diet alone to lose weight. Your efforts will be more effective when you include exercise into your weight-loss program. Figure out the reasons why you may lose interest in your workout routine. Excuses such as *I don't have the time, It's too much work, I don't see a difference,* are counterproductive. Find a solution for each excuse so you don't deviate from your plan. Stay motivated by constantly focusing on the benefits of exercise. Exercise will help you lose weight, make you stronger, and give you more energy. Concentrate on the reasons why you want to get fit, slim, and healthy.

A Breakdown of the Nutritional Facts Label

Nutrition Facts

Serving Size 1 cup (228g)
Servings Per Container 2

Amount per Serving

Calories 250 Calories from Fat 110

	% Daily Value*
Total Fat 12g	**18%**
Saturated Fat 3g	**15%**
Trans Fat 3g	
Cholesterol 30mg	**10%**
Sodium 470mg	**20%**
Total Carbohydrate 31g	**10%**
Dietary Fiber 0g	**0%**
Sugars 5g	
Protein 5g	

Vitamin A	**4%**
Vitamin C	**2%**
Calcium	**20%**
Iron	**4%**

* Percent Daily Values are based on a 2,000 calorie diet.
Your Daily Values may be higher or lower depending on your
calorie needs.

	Calories:	2,000	2,500
Total Fat	Less than	65g	80g
Sat Fat	Less than	20g	25g
Cholesterol	Less than	300mg	300mg
Sodium	Less than	2,400mg	2,400mg
Total Carbohydrate		300g	375g
Dietary Fiber		25g	30g

1
2
3
4
5

The first place to look when selecting foods at the market is the product label. Check out the Nutrition Facts for the ingredient list, serving size, calories, amounts, nutrients, portions, and percentage of daily nutritional values. Often you will see "enriched" food sources for wheat or pasta. This is an indication that vitamins or minerals have been added for nutrition. Commonly added nutrients are calcium, thiamin, riboflavin, niacin, iron, and folic acid. The ingredient list tells you exactly what is in the food, including nutrients and whether fat or sugar have been added. The ingredients are also listed in descending order by weight.

Label at a Glance:
Check the serving size and servings per container.

1. **Calories:** 400 or more calories per serving are considered high. Note the calories from fat.
2. **Daily Values:** 5 percent = low, 20 percent = high. **Nutrients to Limit:** Too much fat, saturated fat, trans fat, cholesterol, and sodium may increase your risk of diseases such as heart disease, some cancers, or high blood pressure.
3. **Get Enough of These Nutrients:** Most Americans do not receive the proper amount of fiber, vitamins A and C, calcium, or iron from their diets. Eating enough of these nutrients can limit your risk of diseases such as osteoporosis and heart disease.
4. **Daily Values Footnote:** This footnote makes recommendations for key nutrients based on diets of 2,000 and 2,500 daily calories.

FATS AND THEIR SOURCES

SATURATED FATS: Tend to raise blood cholesterol. Foods that contain higher amounts of saturated fats include high fat dairy products (like cheese, whole milk, cream, and regular ice cream), butter, fatty meats, lard, palm oil, and coconut oil.

TRANS FATTY ACIDS: Foods that are high in trans fatty acids tend to raise blood cholesterol as well. These foods include those high in partially hydrogenated vegetable oils, such as hard margarine and shortenings. Foods with a high amount of this type of fat include some commercially fried foods and some baked goods.

DIETARY CHOLESTEROL: Foods that are high in cholesterol also tend to raise blood cholesterol. These foods include liver and other organ meats, egg yolks, and dairy fat.

UNSATURATED FATS: Unsaturated fats and oils do not raise blood cholesterol. These types of fats occur in vegetable oils such as olive, canola, and corn oils, most nuts, avocados, and fatty fish like salmon. Some fish, such as salmon, tuna, and mackerel, contain omega-3 fatty acids that may offer protection against heart disease. This is the best type of fat to include in your diet. Just be sure to avoid excess calories.

Best Sources
for Essential Nutrients

BEST SOURCES FOR CALCIUM

Milk & dairy	yogurt, cheese, milk
Seafood	sardines, pink salmon, perch, blue crab, clams
Various vegetables	collard, turnip, and dandelion greens, spinach
Peas/beans/legumes	soybeans/tofu, black-eyed peas, white beans
Fortified foods	cereals, soy milk, oatmeal

BEST SOURCES FOR IRON

Shellfish	clams, oysters, shrimp
Organ meats	liver, giblets
Beans/legumes/peas	soy, white, kidney, lima, navy, lentils
Lean meats	beef, duck, lamb
Various fruit/vegetables	spinach, prune juice, tomato puree/paste

BEST SOURCES FOR VITAMIN A, & VITAMIN C

SOURCES OF VITAMIN A:

Organ meats	liver, giblets

BEST SOURCES FOR VITAMIN A & VITAMIN C

Dark leafy vegetables   collard, turnip, and mustard greens, kale
Orange fruit/vegetables   carrots, sweet potato, pumpkin, squash

SOURCES OF VITAMIN C:
Various fruits   cantaloupe, grapefruit, guava, kiwi, mango, orange, strawberries, papaya, pineapple
Various vegetables   red/green sweet pepper, brussels sprouts, broccoli, sweet potato, cauliflower, kale

BEST SOURCES FOR VITAMIN E & POTASSIUM

SOURCES OF VITAMIN E:
Fortified foods   ready-to-eat cereals
Seeds & nuts   sunflower seeds, almonds, hazelnuts, pine nuts
Oils   sunflower, cottonseed, safflower, canola, peanut

SOURCES OF POTASSIUM:
Various vegetables   sweet potato, tomato puree/paste, beet greens, potato, carrot juice, winter squash, spinach
Beans/legumes/peas   white beans, soybeans, lentils, kidney beans
Milk & dairy   yogurt, milk
Various fruits   prune juice, bananas, peaches, prunes, apricots

CALORIES BURNED FOR TYPICAL PHYSICAL ACTIVITIES

LIGHT ACTIVITIES - 150 or less	CAL/HR.
Billiards	140
Lying down/sleeping	60
Office work	140
Sitting	80
Standing	100

MODERATE ACTIVITIES - 150-350	CAL/HR.
Aerobic dancing	340
Ballroom dancing	210
Bicycling (5 mph)	170
Bowling	160
Canoeing (2.5 mph)	170
Dancing (social)	210
Gardening (moderate)	270
Golf (with cart)	180
Golf (without cart)	320

MODERATE ACTIVITIES - 150-350 (continued)	CAL/HR.
Grocery shopping	180
Horseback riding (sitting trot)	250
Light housework/cleaning, etc.	250
Ping-pong	270
Swimming (20 yards/min)	290
Tennis (recreational doubles)	310
Vacuuming	220
Volleyball (recreational)	260
Walking (2 mph)	200
Walking (3 mph)	240
Walking (4 mph)	300

VIGOROUS ACTIVITIES - 350 or MORE	CAL/HR.
Aerobics (step)	440
Backpacking (10 lb load)	540
Badminton	450
Basketball (competitive)	660
Basketball (leisure)	390
Bicycling (10 mph)	375
Bicycling (13 mph)	600

VIGOROUS ACTIVITIES - 350 or MORE	CAL/HR.
Cross country skiing (leisurely)	460
Cross country skiing (moderate)	660
Hiking	460
Ice skating (9 mph)	384
Jogging (5 mph)	550
Jogging (6 mph)	690
Racquetball	620
Rollerblading	384
Rowing machine	540
Running (8 mph)	900
Scuba diving	570
Shoveling snow	580
Soccer	580
Spinning	650
Stair climber machine	480
Swimming (50 yards/min.)	680
Water aerobics	400
Water skiing	480
Weight training (30 sec. between sets)	760
Weight training (60 sec. between sets)	570

CONCLUSION

By now, you should feel good about your prospects for successfully losing weight and keeping it off. *Simple Principles to Eat Smart and Lose Weight* will help you take charge of your weight loss program. If you follow the hints, tips, ideas, suggestions, and other principles contained in this book, you are closer than ever to achieving your desired weight. Refer back to this book when you feel your weight loss progress stalling or if you decide to set a new goal weight. It is a useful resource for nutritional information, fitness guidelines, weight-loss statistics, and expert advice that will help you successfully lose weight and keep it off.

In addition to reading this book, you should keep a journal of what you eat every single day. Being aware of what you eat is an important step in the direction of weight loss: You should also take photos of yourself as you lose weight so you can track your progress and feel good when you reach important goals.

Along with writing down what you eat in a food journal, keep an exercise journal that charts the amount of activity you get every single day. Mark how long you ran on the treadmill at the gym; how many reps and arm curls you did; how many calories your pedometer says you burned on your morning walk; and other activities that help you lose weight.

Keeping track of your calorie intake along with your exercise program will keep you motivated to maintain your weight-loss goal.

With *Simple Principles to Eat Smart and Lose Weight* as your companion, you will make wiser, more informed choices that will help you lose weight, look better, and improve your health. Practice what you have learned in this book often. Keep it handy and refer to it when you need a reminder. The key thing to remember is that losing weight is completely within your reach if you follow all of the suggestions made in this book. Congratulations on your weight loss accomplishments!

NUTRITIONAL INFORMATION

Nutrition values for fat, protein, carbohydrates, and fiber are listed in grams per serving.
Serving sizes and values are approximate.

FOOD ITEM	Serving Size	Cal.	Fat	Protein	Carbs	Fiber
A						
Alcohol, 100 proof	1 fl oz	82	0	0	0	0
Alcohol, 86 proof	1 fl oz	70	0	0	0	0
Alcohol, 90 proof	1 fl oz	73	0	0	0	0
Alcohol, 94 proof	1 fl oz	76	0	0	0	0
Alcohol, dessert wine, dry	1 glass	157	0	0.2	12	0
Alcohol, dessert wine, sweet	1 glass	165	0	0.2	14.1	0
Alcohol, liquors	1 fl oz	107	0.1	0	11.2	0
Alcohol, pina colada	8 fl oz	440	4.8	1	57	0.4
Alfalfa seeds	1 tbsp	1	0	0.1	0.1	0.1
Allspice, ground	1 tsp	5	0.2	0.1	1.4	0.4
Almond butter, w/ salt	1 tbsp	101	9.5	2.4	3.4	0.6
Almond butter, w/o salt	1 tbsp	101	9.5	2.4	3.4	0.6
Almonds, roasted	1 oz (12 nuts)	169	15	6.2	5.5	3.3
Anchovies	3 oz	111	4.1	17.3	0	0
Apple cider, powdered	1 packet	83	0	0	20.7	0
Apple juice	8 fl oz	120	0.2	0.2	28.8	0
Apples, w/o skin	1 medium	61	0.2	0.3	16	1.7
Apples, w/ skin	1 medium	72	0.2	0.4	19	3.3
Applesauce	1 cup	194	0.5	0.5	50.8	3.1
Apricots	1 apricot	17	0.1	0.5	3.9	0.7
Arrowroot	1 cup, sliced	78	0.2	5.1	16.1	1.6
Arrowroot flour	1 cup	457	0.1	0.4	112.8	4.4
Artichokes	1 artichoke	76	0.2	5.3	17	8.7
Arugula	1 cup	4	0.1	0.5	0.7	0.4
Asparagus	1 spear	2	0	0.3	0.5	0.3
Avocados	1 cup, cubes	240	22	3	12.8	10
B						
Bacon bits, meatless	1 tbsp	33	1.8	2.2	2	0.7

FOOD ITEM	Serving Size	Cal.	Fat	Protein	Carbs	Fiber
B (cont.)						
Bacon, canadian, cooked	1 slice	43	2	5.8	0.3	0
Bacon, meatless	1 slice	16	1.5	0.5	0.3	0.1
Bacon, pork, cooked	1 slice	42	3.2	3	0.1	0
Bagels, cinnamon-raisin	1 bagel, 4" dia	244	1.5	8.7	49	2
Bagels, egg	1 bagel, 4" dia	292	2.2	11	55.6	2.4
Bagels, oat-bran	1 bagel, 4" dia	227	1	9.5	47	3.2
Bagels, plain	1 bagel, 4" dia	245	1.4	9.3	47	2
Bagels, deli gourmet style	1 bagel	370	3	13	71	2
Balsam pear	1 balsam pear	21	0.2	1.2	4.6	3.5
Bamboo shoots	1 cup	41	0.5	3.9	7.9	3.3
Banana chips	1 oz.	147	9.5	0.7	16.6	2.2
Bananas	1 medium, 7"-8"	105	0.4	13	27	3
Barley	1 cup	651	4.2	23	135.2	31.8
Barley flour	1 cup	511	2.4	15.5	110.3	14.9
Barley, pearled, cooked	1 cup	193	0.7	3.6	44.3	6
Basil	5 leaves	1	0	0.1	0.1	0.1
Basil, dried	1 tsp.	2	0	0.1	0.4	0.3
Bay leaf	1 tsp, crumbled	2	0.1	0	0.4	0.2
Beans, adzuki, cooked	1 cup	294	0.2	17	57	16.8
Beans, baked, canned, plain	1 cup	239	0.9	12.1	53.7	10.4
Beans, baked, canned, w/o salt	1 cup	266	1	12.1	52.1	13.9
Beans, baked, canned, w/ beef	1 cup	322	9.2	17	45	10
Beans, black, cooked	1 cup	227	0.9	15	40	15
Beans, cranberry, cooked	1 cup	241	0.8	16	43	18
Beans, fava, canned	1 cup	182	0.5	14	31	9.5
Beans, french, cooked	1 cup	228	1.3	12	43	17
Beans, great northern, cooked	1 cup	209	0.8	15	37	12
Beans, kidney, cooked	1 cup	225	0.9	15	40	11
Beans, lima, cooked	1 cup	216	0.7	15	39	13
Beans, lima, canned	1 can	190	0.4	12	36	11
Beans, mung, cooked	1 cup	212	0.7	14	39	15
Beans, mungo, cooked	1 cup	189	1	13.5	33	11.5
Beans, navy, cooked	1 cup	255	1	15	47	19
Beans, pink, cooked	1 cup	252	0.8	15	47	9

FOOD ITEM	Serving Size	Cal.	Fat	Protein	Carbs	Fiber

B (cont.)

FOOD ITEM	Serving Size	Cal.	Fat	Protein	Carbs	Fiber
Beans, pinto, cooked	1 cup	245	1	15	44	15
Beans, small white, cooked	1 cup	254	1	16	46	18
Beans, snap, green, cooked	1 cup	44	0.3	2	10	4
Beans, snap, yellow, cooked	1 cup	44	0.3	2	10	4
Beans, white, cooked	1 cup	249	0.6	17	45	11
Beans, yellow	1 cup	255	2	16	48	18
Beechnuts, dried	1 oz	163	14.2	1.8	9.5	0
Beef, choice short rib, cooked	3 oz	400	35.6	18.3	0	0
Beef bologna	1 slice	88	8	3.3	0.6	0
Beef jerky, chopped	1 piece	81	5.1	6.6	2.2	0.4
Beef sausage, precooked	1 link	134	11.6	6	1	0
Beef stew, canned	1 serving	218	12.5	11.5	15.7	3.5
Beef, tri-tip roast, roasted	3 oz	174	9.4	22.2	0	0
Beef, brisket, lean and fat, roasted	3 oz	328	26.8	20	0	0
Beef, brisket, lean, roasted	3 oz	206	10.8	25.3	0	0
Beef, chuck, arm roast, lean & fat, braised	3 oz	283	19.6	23.3	0	0
Beef, chuck, arm roast, lean, braised	3 oz	179	6.5	28.1	0	0
Beef, chuck, top blade, raw	3 oz	138	7.5	16.5	0	0
Beef, cured breakfast strips	3 slices	276	26.4	8.5	0.5	0
Beef, cured, corned, canned	3 oz	213	12.8	23	0	0
Beef, cured, dried	1 serving	43	0.5	8.7	0.8	0
Beef, cured, luncheon meat	1 slice	31	0.9	5.4	0	0
Beef, flank, raw	1 oz	47	2.4	6	0	0
Beef, ground patties, frozen	3 oz	240	19.7	14.5	0	0
Beef, ground, 70% lean, raw	1 oz	94	8.5	4.1	0	0
Beef, ground, 80% lean, raw	1 oz	72	5.7	4.9	0	0
Beef, ground, 95% lean, raw	1 oz	39	1.4	6.1	0	0
Beef, rib, large end, boneless, raw	1 oz	94	8.3	4.5	0	0
Beef, rib, shortribs, boneless, raw	1 oz	110	10.3	4.1	0	0
Beef, rib, whole, boneless, raw	1 oz	91	7.9	4.6	0	0
Beef, rib-eye, small end, raw	1 oz	78	6.3	5	0	0
Beef, round, bottom, raw	1 oz	56	3.4	5.9	0	0
Beef, round, eye, raw	1 oz	49	2.5	6.1	0	0
Beef, round, full cut, raw	1 oz	55	3.4	5.8	0	0

FOOD ITEM	Serving Size	Cal.	Fat	Protein	Carbs	Fiber
B (cont.)						
Beef, round, tip, raw	1 oz	56	3.6	5.5	0	0
Beef, round, top, raw	1 oz	48	2.3	6.2	0	0
Beef, shank crosscuts, raw	1 oz	50	2.8	5.8	0	0
Beef, short loin, porterhouse, raw	1 oz	73	5.7	5.1	0	0
Beef, short loin, t-bone, raw	1 oz	66	4.8	5.4	0	0
Beef, short loin, top, raw	1 oz	66	4.5	5.8	0	0
Beef, sirloin, tri-tip, raw	1 oz	50	3	5.8	0	0
Beef, tenderloin, raw	1 oz	70	5.1	5.6	0	0
Beef, top sirloin, raw	1 oz	61	4	5.6	0	0
Beer, light	12 fl oz	110	12	4.8	7	0
Beer, nonalcoholic	12 fl oz	80	1	0	70	0
Beer, regular	12 fl oz	140	12	0.9	10	0.7
Beets	1 beet	35	0	2	8	4
Bratwurst, chicken	1 serving	148	8.7	16.3	0	0
Bratwurst, pork	1 serving	281	24.8	11.7	2.1	0
Bratwurst, veal	1 serving	286	26.6	11.8	0	0
Bread stuffing, dry mix, prepared	1/2 cup	178	8.6	3	22	3
Bread, banana	1 slice	196	6.3	2.5	32.7	0.7
Bread, corn	1 piece	188	6	4.3	28.8	1.4
Bread, cracked-wheat	1 slice	65	1	2.2	11.8	1
Bread, french	1 slice	70	1	3	15	1
Bread, garlic	1 slice	160	10	3	14	1
Bread, Irish soda	1 oz	82	1.4	1.9	15.9	0.7
Bread, pita	2 oz	150	1	3	30	0
Bread, pumpernickel	1 slice	75	1	3	15	2
Bread, raisin	1 slice	80	1.5	2	15	1
Bread, rice bran	1 oz	69	1.3	2.5	12.3	1.4
Bread, sandwich slice	1 slice	70	1	2	13	1
Bread, sourdough	1 slice	100	1	2	20	1
Broad beans, cooked	1 cup	187	0.6	13	33.4	9.2
Brownies	1 brownie	220	13	1	27	1
Buckwheat	1 cup	583	5.8	22.5	121.6	17
Buckwheat flour	1 cup	402	3.7	15.1	84.7	12
Buckwheat groats, roasted, cooked	1 cup	155	1	5.6	33.5	4.5

FOOD ITEM	Serving Size	Cal.	Fat	Protein	Carbs	Fiber
Buffalo, raw	1 oz.	28	0.4	5.8	0	0
Burbot, raw	3 oz.	77	0.7	16.4	0	0
Burdock root	1 cup	85	0.2	1.8	20.5	3.9
Butter, whipped, w/ salt	1 tbsp.	67	7.6	0.1	0	0
Butternuts, dried	1 oz.	174	16	7	3	1.3

C

FOOD ITEM	Serving Size	Cal.	Fat	Protein	Carbs	Fiber
Cabbage, common	1 cup, shredded	17	1	1	4	1.6
Cabbage, pak choi	1 cup, shredded	9	0.1	1.1	1.5	0.7
Cabbage, pe-tsai	1 cup, shredded	12	0.2	0.9	2.5	0.9
Cake, angel food	1 slice	180	4	2	36	2
Cake, boston cream pie	1 slice	260	9	1	32	0
Cake, carrot	1 slice	310	16	1	39	0
Cake, cheesecake	1 slice	500	30	4	50	0
Cake, chocolate	1 slice	270	13	1	36	1
Cake, chocolate mousse	1 slice	250	10	1	35	1
Cake, devil's food	1 slice	270	13	2	35	0
Cake, pineapple upside-down	1 piece	367	13.9	4	58.1	0.9
Cake, pound	1 slice	320	16	2	38	0
Cake, sponge cake w/ cream, berries	1 slice	325	8	25	38	1
Cake, yellow	1 slice	260	11	2	36	1
Candy, butterscotch	5 pieces	120	2.5	0	20	0
Candy, caramels	1 piece	30	1	3	6	1
Candy, carob	1 bar	470	27.3	7.1	49	3.3
Candy, chocolate fudge	1 oz.	125	5	0	18	0
Candy, chocolate mints	1 mint	45	1	0	9	0
Candy, milk chocolate w/ almonds	1.5 oz.	216	14	3.7	21	2.5
Candy, chocolate-coated peanut butter bites	1 piece	45	2.5	1	4	0
Candy, chocolate-coated peanuts	12 peanuts	160	11	20	15	7
Candy, gumdrops	4 pieces	130	0	0	31	0
Candy, hard candy	1 piece	18	0	0	5	0
Candy, jelly beans	12 beans	100	0	0	24	0
Candy, licorice	1 piece	30	0	0	7	0
Candy, lollipop	1 lollipop	20	0	0	5	0
Candy, milk chocolate bar	1.5 oz.	235	13	3.3	26	1.5

FOOD ITEM	Serving Size	Cal.	Fat	Protein	Carbs	Fiber
C (cont.)						
Candy, mints	1 mint	30	0	0	7	0
Cantaloupe	1 cup, cubed	54	0.3	1.3	13.1	1.4
Cardoon	1 cup, shredded	36	0.2	1.2	8.7	2.8
Carrots	1 medium	65	0	1	15	4
Cashew butter, w/ salt	1 tbsp	94	7.9	2.8	4.4	0.3
Cashew nuts	1 oz	157	12.4	5.2	8.6	0.9
Cassava	1 cup	330	0.6	2.8	78.4	3.7
Celeraic	1 cup	66	0.5	2.3	14.4	2.8
Chard, swiss	1 cup	7	0.1	0.6	1.3	0.6
Cheese, american	1 slice	110	9	5	1	0
Cheese, brick	1 oz	100	8	31	0	0
Cheese, brie	1 oz	95	8	50	1	0
Cheese, camembert	1 oz	90	7	49	1	0
Cheese, cheddar	1 oz	110	9	33	0.5	0
Cheese, colby jack	1 oz	110	9	31	0.5	0
Cheese, cottage, 2%	1 cup	203	4	31	8	0
Cheese, edam	1 oz	100	8	7	0	0
Cheese, feta	1 oz	100	8	21	1	0
Cheese, goat	1 oz	128	10.1	8.7	0.6	0
Cheese, goat, semisoft	1 oz	103	8.5	6.1	0.7	0
Cheese, goat, soft	1 oz	76	6	5.3	0.3	0
Cheese, gouda	1 oz	100	8	7	0.5	0
Cheese, monterey jack	1 oz	110	9	32	0	0
Cheese, mozzarella	1 oz	90	7	25	0.5	0
Cheese, parmesan, hard	1 oz	110	7	10	1	0
Cheese, parmesan, shredded	1 tbsp	22	1.5	2	0	0
Cheese, provolone	1 oz	100	8	34	1	0
Cheese, queso	2 tbsp	110	9	28	2	0
Cheese, ricotta	2 tbsp	50	3.5	28	1	0
Cheese, roquefort	1 oz	105	9	6	0.5	0
Cheese, swiss	1 oz	110	9	36	1	0
Cherries, sour	8 pieces	30	0	1	7	2
Cherries, sweet	8 pieces	30	0	2	7	2
Chewing gum	1 piece	25	0	0	5	0

FOOD ITEM

FOOD ITEM	Serving Size	Cal.	Fat	Protein	Carbs	Fiber

C (cont.)

FOOD ITEM	Serving Size	Cal.	Fat	Protein	Carbs	Fiber
Chicken, breast, w/ skin	1/2 breast	249	13.4	30.2	0	0
Chicken, breast, w/o skin	1/2 breast	130	1.5	27.2	0	0
Chicken, capons, boneless	1/2 capon	1459	74	184	0	0
Chicken, capons, giblets, cooked	1 cup	238	8	38	1	0
Chicken, cornish game hen, roasted	1/2 bird	336	24	29	0	0
Chicken, cornish game hen, meat only	1 bird	295	9	51	0	0
Chicken, dark meat, w/o skin	1 cup diced	287	14	38	0	0
Chicken, drumstick, w/ skin	1 drumstick	118	6.3	14.1	0	0
Chicken, drumstick, w/o skin	1 drumstick	74	2.1	12.8	0	0
Chicken, leg, w/ skin	1 leg	312	20.2	30.3	0	0
Chicken, leg, w/o skin	1 leg	156	5	26.2	0	0
Chicken, light meat, w/o skin	1 cup diced	214	6	38	0	0
Chicken, thigh, w/ skin	1 thigh	198	14.3	16.2	0	0
Chicken, thigh, w/o skin	1 thigh	82	2.7	13.6	0	0
Chicken, wing, w/ skin	1 wing	109	7.8	9	0	0
Chicken, wing, w/o skin	1 wing	37	1	6.4	0	0
Chickpeas, cooked	1 cup	269	4	15	45	12.5
Chicory greens	1 cup, chopped	41	0.5	3.1	8.5	7.2
Chicory roots	1/2 cup	33	0.1	0.6	7.9	0
Chicory, witloof	1/2 cup	8	0	0.4	1.8	1.4
Chili con carne w/ beans	1 cup	298	13	17.5	28	10
Chili powder	1 tsp	8	0.4	0.3	1.4	0.9
Chili w/ beans, canned	1 cup	287	14	14.5	30.5	11
Chili w/o beans, canned	1 cup	194	6.5	17	18	3
Chinese chestnuts	1 oz	64	0.3	1.2	13.9	0
Chives	1 tbsp, chopped	1	0	0.1	0.1	0.1
Chocolate chip crisped rice bar	1 bar	115	3.8	1.4	20.7	0.6
Chocolate chips	1/4 cup	210	12	3	24	1
Chocolate milk shake, ready-to-drink	8 fl oz	181	5	8	26	1
Chocolate, semi sweet bars, baking	1 oz	160	8	3	20	1
Chocolate, unsweetened baking squares	1 square	144	15	3.7	8.6	4.8
Chorizo, pork and beef	1 link	273	23	14.5	1.1	0
Chow mein noodles	1 cup	237	13.8	3.8	25.9	1.8
Cinnamon, ground	1 tsp	6	0.1	0.1	1.8	1.2

FOOD ITEM	Serving Size	Cal.	Fat	Protein	Carbs	Fiber

C (cont.)

FOOD ITEM	Serving Size	Cal.	Fat	Protein	Carbs	Fiber
Cisco	3 oz	83	1.6	16.1	0	0
Citrus fruit drink, from concentrate	8 fl oz	124	0.1	0.5	30	0.8
Clam, mixed species, raw	1 large	15	0.2	2.6	0.5	0
Cloves, ground	1 tsp	7	0.4	0.1	1.3	0.7
Cocktail mix, nonalcoholic	1 fl oz	103	0	0.1	25.8	0
Cocoa mix, powder	1 serving	113	1.1	1.7	24	1
Cocoa mix, powder, unsweetened	1 tbsp	12	0.7	1.1	2.9	1.8
Coconut meat	1 cup, shredded	283	26.8	2.7	12.2	7.2
Coconut milk	1 cup	552	57.2	5.5	13.3	5.3
Coffee, brewed, decaf	1 cup	0	0	0.2	0	0
Coffee, brewed, regular	1 cup	2	0	0.3	0	0
Coffee, café au lait	8 fl oz	65	2.5	1	6	0
Coffee, cappuccino	8 fl oz	70	4	1	6	0
Coffee, espresso	1 shot	4	0	0	1	0
Coffee, instant, decaf	1 tsp	0	0	0	0	0
Coffee, instant, regular	1 tsp, dry	2	0	0.1	0.4	0
Coffee, latte	8 fl oz	100	5	0	8	0
Coffee, mocha	8 fl oz	180	12	1	16	0*
Coffee cake	2.5 oz	230	7	3.8	38	3.8
Coleslaw	1/2 cup	41	1.6	0.8	7.4	0.9
Collards	1 cup, chopped	11	0.2	0.9	2	1.3
Conch, baked or broiled	1 cup, sliced	165	1.5	33.4	2.2	0
Cookies, animal crackers	1 cookie	22	0.7	0.3	3.6	0.1
Cookies, brownies	3.5 oz	430	25	1	52	1.2
Cookies, butter	1 cookie	23	0.9	0.3	3.4	0
Cookies, chocolate chip, deli fresh baked	1 cookie	275	15	0	37.5	1
Cookies, chocolate chip, commercial	1 cookie	130	6.9	0.9	16.7	0.9
Cookies, chocolate chip, refrigerated dough	1 portion	128	5.9	1.3	17.8	0.4
Cookies, chocolate wafers	1 wafer	26	0.8	0.4	4.3	0.2
Cookies, fig bars	1 cookie	150	3.1	1.6	30.5	2
Cookies, fudge	1 cookie	73	0.8	1.1	16.4	0.6
Cookies, gingersnap	1 cookie	29	0.7	0.4	5.4	0.2
Cookies, graham, plain or honey	2 1/2" square	30	0.7	0.5	5.3	0.2
Cookies, marshmallow w/ chocolate coating	1 cookie	118	4.7	1.1	19	0.6

C (cont.)

FOOD ITEM	Serving Size	Cal.	Fat	Protein	Carbs	Fiber
Cookies, molasses	1 cookie	138	4.1	1.8	23.6	0.3
Cookies, oatmeal	1 cookie	238	8.8	2.5	37.5	2
Cookies, oatmeal w/ raisins	1 cookie	238	8.8	2.5	37.5	2
Cookies, oatmeal, commercial, iced	1 cookie	123	4.8	1.4	18.4	0.6
Cookies, oatmeal, refrigerated dough	1 portion	68	3	0.9	9.5	0.4
Cookies, peanut butter sandwich	1 cookie	67	3	1.2	9.2	0.3
Cookies, peanut butter, refrigerated dough	1 portion	73	4	1.3	8.3	0.2
Cookies, sugar	1 cookie	66	3.3	0.8	8.4	0.2
Cookies, sugar wafers w/ cream filling	1 wafer	46	2.2	0.4	6.3	0.1
Cookies, sugar, refrigerated dough	1 portion	113	5.4	1.1	15.3	0.2
Cookies, vanilla wafers	1 wafer	28	1.2	0.3	4.3	0.1
Coriander leaves	9 sprigs	5	0.1	0.4	0.7	0.6
Corn flour, yellow	1 cup	416	4.3	10.6	86.9	0
Corn, sweet, white	1 ear	77	1.1	2.9	17.1	2.4
Corn, sweet, yellow	1 ear	77	1.1	2.9	17.1	2.4
Corn, sweet, white, cream style	1 cup	184	1	4.5	46.4	3.1
Corn, sweet, yellow, cream style	1 cup	184	1	4.5	46.4	3.1
Cornnuts	1 oz	126	4.4	2.4	20.4	2
Cornstarch	1 cup	488	0.1	0.3	116.8	1.2
Couscous, cooked	1 cup	176	0.2	6	36.5	0.1
Cowpeas (black-eyed peas), cooked	1 cup	160	0.6	5.2	33.5	8.2
Cowpeas, catjang, cooked	1 cup	200	1.2	14	34.7	6.2
Cowpeas, leafy tips	1 cup, chopped	10	0.1	1.5	1.7	0
Crab, alaska king, raw	1 leg	144	1	31.5	0	0
Crab, blue, canned	1 cup	134	1.6	27.7	0	0
Crab, dungeness, cooked	1 crab	140	1.6	28.4	1.2	0
Crabapples	1 cup, sliced	84	0.3	0.4	21.9	0
Crackers w/ cheese filling	6 crackers	191	9.5	3.5	22.9	0.7
Crackers w/ peanut butter filling	6 cracker	193	9.8	4.8	22.1	1.3
Crackers, cheese, regular	6 crackers	312	15.7	6.3	36.1	1.5
Crackers, graham	1 cracker	30	0.5	6	5	2
Crackers, matzo, plain	1 matzo	112	0.4	2.8	23.7	0.9
Crackers, matzo, whole-wheat	1 matzo	100	0.4	3.7	22.4	3.3
Crackers, melba toast	1 cup	129	1.1	4	25.3	2.1

C (cont.)

FOOD ITEM	Serving Size	Cal.	Fat	Protein	Carbs	Fiber
Crackers, milk	1 cracker	50	1.7	0.8	7.7	0.2
Crackers, regular	1 cup, bite size	311	15.7	4.6	37.8	1
Crackers, rusk toast	1 rusk	41	0.7	1.4	7.2	0
Crackers, rye	1 cracker	37	0.1	1.1	8.8	2.5
Crackers, saltines	1 cracker	20	0.1	0.5	4.1	0.1
Crackers, soda	1 cracker	60	2	6	10	2
Crackers, wheat	1 cracker	9	0.4	0.1	1.3	0.1
Crackers, wheat, sandwich w/ peanut butter	1 cracker	35	1.8	0.9	3.7	0.3
Crackers, whole-wheat	1 cracker	18	0.7	0.3	2.7	0.4
Cranberries	1 cup, whole	44	0.1	0.4	11.6	4.4
Cranberry juice cocktail	1 cup	144	0.3	0	36.4	0.3
Cranberry-apple juice	1 cup	174	0.1	0.2	44.3	0.2
Cranberry-grape juice	1 cup	137	0.2	0.5	34.3	0.2
Crayfish, wild, raw	8 crayfish	21	0.3	4.3	0	0
Cream cheese	1 tbsp.	51	5.1	1.1	0.4	0
Cream of tartar	1 tsp.	8	0	0	1.8	0
Cream, half & half	1 tbsp.	20	1.7	0.4	0.6	0
Cream, heavy whipping	1 cup, fluid	821	88.1	4.9	6.6	0
Crepes	1 crepe	120	6	2	14	1
Croissants, apple	1 croissant	145	5	4.2	21.1	1.4
Croissants, butter	1 croissant	115	6	2.3	13	0.7
Croissants, cheese	1 croissant	174	8.8	3.9	19.7	1.1
Croutons, plain	1 cup	122	2	3.6	22.1	1.5
Croutons, seasoned	1 cup	186	7.3	4.3	25.4	2
Cucumber	1 cucumber	45	0.3	2	10.9	1.5
Cucumber, peeled	1 cup, sliced	14	0.2	0.7	2.6	0.8
Cumin seed	1 tsp.	8	0.5	0.4	0.9	0.2
Currants, black	1 cup	71	0.5	1.6	17.2	0
Currants, red & white	1 cup	63	0.2	1.6	15.5	4.8
Curry powder	1 tsp.	7	0.3	0.3	1.2	0.7

D

FOOD ITEM	Serving Size	Cal.	Fat	Protein	Carbs	Fiber
Dandelion greens	1 cup, chopped	25	0.4	1.5	5.1	1.9
Danish pastry, cheese, 4 1/4" diameter	1 pastry	266	15.5	5.7	26.4	0.7

FOOD ITEM	Serving Size	Cal.	Fat	Protein	Carbs	Fiber
D (cont.)						
Danish pastry, cinnamon, 4 1/4" diameter	1 pastry	262	14.5	4.5	29	0.8
Danish pastry, fruit, 4 1/4" diameter	1 pastry	263	13	3.8	33.9	1.3
Danish pastry, nut, 4 1/4" diameter	1 pastry	280	16.4	4.6	29.7	1.3
Danish pastry, raspberry, 4 1/4" diameter	1 pastry	263	13.1	3.8	33.9	1.3
Deer, ground, raw	1 oz.	45	2	6.2	0	0
Deer, raw	1 oz.	34	0.7	6.5	0	0
Doughnuts, chocolate coated or frosted	1 doughnut	133	8.7	1.4	13.4	0.6
Doughnuts, chocolate, sugared or glazed	1 doughnut	250	11.9	2.7	34.4	1.3
Doughnuts, french crullers	1 cruller	169	7.5	1.3	24.4	0.5
Doughnuts, plain	1 doughnut, stick	219	11.9	2.6	25.8	0.8
Doughnuts, wheat, sugared or glazed	1 doughnut	101	5.4	1.8	11.9	0.6
Duck liver, raw	1 liver	60	2	8.2	1.6	0
Duck, meat only, roasted	1/2 duck	444	24.7	51.9	0	0
Duck, white pekin, breast w/skin, roasted	1/2 breast	242	13	29.4	0	0
Duck, skinless, raw	1/2 duck	400	18	55.4	0	0
Durian	1 cup, chopped	357	13	3.6	65.8	9.2
E						
Eclairs w/ chocolate glaze	1 éclair	293	17.6	7.2	27.1	0.7
Eel, mixed species, raw	3 oz.	156	9.9	15.7	0	0
Egg noodles, cooked	1 cup	213	2.3	7.6	39.7	1.8
Egg substitute, liquid	1 tbsp.	13	0.5	1.9	0.1	0
Egg white, fried	1 large	92	7	6.3	0.4	0
Egg white, raw	1 large	17	0.1	3.6	0.2	0
Egg yolk, raw	1 large	53	4.4	2.6	0.6	0
Egg, hard-boiled	1 cup, chopped	211	14.4	17.1	1.5	0
Egg, omelette	1 large	93	7.3	6.5	0.4	0
Egg, poached	1 large	74	4.9	6.3	0.4	0
Egg, raw	1 large	85	5.8	7.3	0.4	0
Egg, scrambled	1 cup	365	26.9	24.4	4.8	0
Eggnog	8 fl oz.	343	19	9.6	34	0
Eggplant	1 eggplant	110	0.9	4.6	26.1	15.6
Elderberries	1 cup	106	0.7	1	26.7	10.2
Elk, ground, raw	1 oz.	49	2.5	6.2	0	0

FOOD ITEM	Serving Size	Cal.	Fat	Protein	Carbs	Fiber
E (cont.)						
Elk, raw	1 oz	31	0.4	6.5	0	0
Endive	1 head	87	1	6.4	17.2	15.9
English muffins, plain	1 muffin	134	1	4.4	26.2	1.5
English muffins, cinnamon-raisin	1 muffin	139	1.5	4.2	48.7	1.7
English muffins, wheat	1 muffin	127	1.1	5	25.5	2.6
English muffins, whole-wheat	1 muffin	134	1.4	5.8	26.6	4.4
English muffins, whole-wheat/multigrain	1 muffin	155	1.2	6	30.5	1.8
European chestnuts, peeled	1 oz	56	0.4	0.5	12.5	0
European chestnuts, unpeeled	1 oz	60	0.6	0.7	12.9	2.3
F						
Farina, cooked	1 cup	471	0.1	3.3	24.4	0.7
Fast food, biscuit w/ egg	1 biscuit	373	22.1	11.6	31.9	0.8
Fast food, biscuit w/ egg & bacon	1 biscuit	458	31.1	17	28.6	0.8
Fast food, biscuit w/ egg, bacon & cheese	1 biscuit	477	31.4	16.3	33.4	0.1
Fast food, biscuit w/ sausage	1 biscuit	485	31.8	12.1	40	1.4
Fast food, caramel sundae	1 sundae	304	9.3	7.3	49.3	0
Fast food, cheeseburger, large, double patty	1 sandwich	704	43.7	38	39.7	1
Fast food, cheeseburger, large, single patty	1 sandwich	563	32.9	28.2	38.4	1
Fast food, corndog	1 corndog	460	18.9	16.8	55.8	1
Fast food, croissant w/ egg, cheese	1 croissant	368	24.7	12.8	24.3	1
Fast food, croissant w/ egg, cheese, bacon	1 croissant	413	28.4	16.2	23.6	1
Fast food, croissant w/ egg, cheese, sausage	1 croissant	523	38.2	20.3	24.7	1
Fast food, Danish pastry, cheese	1 pastry	353	24.6	5.8	28.7	1.5
Fast food, Danish pastry, cinnamon	1 pastry	349	16.7	4.8	46.9	1.5
Fast food, Danish pastry, fruit	1 pastry	335	15.9	4.8	45.1	1.5
Fast food, fish sandwich w/ tartar sauce	1 sandwich	431	22.8	16.9	41	1
Fast food, french toast sticks	5 pieces	513	29	8.3	57.9	2.7
Fast food, fried chicken, boneless	6 pieces	285	18.1	15	15.7	0.9
Fast food, hamburger, large, double patty	1 sandwich	540	26.6	34.3	40.3	2.1
Fast food, hamburger, large, single patty	1 sandwich	425	20.9	23	36.7	2.1
Fast food, hot fudge sundae	1 sundae	284	8.6	5.6	47.7	0
Fast food, hot dog w/ chili	1 hot dog	296	13.4	13.5	31.3	1
Fast food, hot dog, plain	1 hot dog	242	14.5	10.4	18	1

FOOD ITEM	Serving Size	Cal.	Fat	Protein	Carbs	Fiber
F (cont.)						
Fast food, McDonald's Big Mac® w/ cheese	1 serving	560	30	25	46	3.1
Fast food, McDonald's Big Mac® w/o cheese	1 serving	495	25.4	23.2	43.3	2.7
Fast food, McDonald's cheeseburger	1 serving	310	12	15	35	1
Fast food, McDonald's Chicken McGrill®	1 serving	400	16	27	38	3
Fast food, McDonald's Crispy Chicken	1 serving	500	23	24	50	3
Fast food, McDonald's Filet-o-Fish®	1 serving	400	18	14	42	1
Fast food, McDonald's french fries	1 medium	350	11	4	47	5
Fast food, McDonald's hamburger	1 serving	260	9	13	33	1
Fast food, McDonald's 1/4 Pounder®,cheese	1 serving	510	25	29	43	3
Fast food, McDonald's 1/4 Pounder®	1 serving	420	18	24	40	3
Fast food, onion rings, 8-9 rings	1 portion	276	15.5	3.7	31.3	3.3
Fast food, strawberry sundae	1 sundae	268	7.8	6.3	44.6	0
Fast food, submarine sandwich w/ cold cuts	1 submarine 6"	456	18.6	21.8	51	4
Fast food, submarine sandwich w/ roast beef	1 submarine 6"	410	13	28.6	44.3	4
Fast food, submarine sandwich w/ tuna	1 submarine 6"	584	28	29.7	55.4	4
Fast food, vanilla soft-serve w/ cone	1 cone	164	6.1	3.9	24.1	0.1
Fennel bulb	1 cup, sliced	27	0.2	1.1	6.3	2.7
Fennel seed	1 tbsp.	20	0.9	0.9	3	2.3
Fenugreek seed	1 tbsp.	36	0.7	2.6	6.5	2.7
Figs	1 medium	37	0.2	0.4	9.6	1.5
Figs, dried	1 fig	21	0.01	0.3	5.3	0.8
Fireweed leaves	1 cup, chopped	24	0.6	1.1	4.4	2.4
Fish oil, cod liver	1 tbsp.	123	13.6	0	0	0
Fish oil, herring	1 tbsp.	123	13.6	0	0	0
Fish oil, menhaden	1 tbsp.	123	13.6	0	0	0
Fish oil, salmon	1 tbsp.	123	13.6	0	0	0
Fish oil, sardine	1 tbsp.	123	13.6	0	0	0
Fish, bluefin tuna, raw	3 oz	122	4.2	19.8	0	0
Fish, bluefish, raw	3 oz	105	3.6	17	0	0
Fish, butterfish, raw	3 oz	124	6.8	14.7	0	0
Fish, carp, raw	3 oz	108	4.8	15.2	0	0
Fish, catfish, raw	3 oz	81	2.4	13.9	0	0
Fish, cod, atlantic, raw	3 oz	70	0.6	15.1	0	0
Fish, croaker, atlantic, raw	3 oz	88	2.7	15.1	0	0

FOOD ITEM

FOOD ITEM	Serving Size	Cal.	Fat	Protein	Carbs	Fiber
F (cont.)						
Fish, flatfish, raw	3 oz.	77	1	16	0	0
Fish, gefilte fish	1 piece	35	0.7	3.8	3.1	0
Fish, grouper, mixed species, raw	3 oz.	78	0.9	16.5	0	0
Fish, haddock, raw	3 oz.	74	0.6	16.1	0	0
Fish, halibut, raw	3 oz.	94	1.9	17.7	0	0
Fish, herring, atlantic, raw	3 oz.	134	7.7	15.3	0	0
Fish, herring, pacific, raw	3 oz.	166	11.8	13.9	0	0
Fish, mackerel, atlantic, raw	3 oz.	174	11.8	15.8	0	0
Fish, mackerel, king, raw	3 oz.	89	1.7	17.2	0	0
Fish, mackerel, pacific, raw	3 oz.	134	6.7	17.1	0	0
Fish, mackerel, spanish, raw	3 oz.	118	5.4	16.4	0	0
Fish, milkfish, raw	3 oz.	126	5.7	17.5	0	0
Fish, monkfish, raw	3 oz.	65	1.3	12.3	0	0
Fish, ocean perch, atlantic, raw	3 oz.	80	1.4	15.8	0	0
Fish, perch, mixed species, raw	3 oz.	77	0.8	16.5	0	0
Fish, pike, northern, raw	3 oz.	75	0.6	16.4	0	0
Fish, pollock, atlantic, raw	3 oz.	78	0.8	16.5	0	0
Fish, pout, ocean, raw	3 oz.	67	0.8	14.1	0	0
Fish, rainbow smelt, raw	3 oz.	82	2.1	15	0	0
Fish, rockfish, pacific, raw	3 oz.	80	1.3	15.9	0	0
Fish, roe, mixed species, raw	1 tbsp.	20	0.9	3.1	0.2	0
Fish, sablefish, raw	3 oz.	166	13	11.4	0	0
Fish, salmon, atlantic, farmed, raw	3 oz.	156	9.2	16.9	0	0
Fish, salmon, atlantic, wild, raw	3 oz.	121	5.4	16.9	0	0
Fish, salmon, chinook, raw	3 oz.	152	8.9	16.9	0	0
Fish, salmon, pink, raw	3 oz.	99	2.9	16.9	0	0
Fish, sea bass, mixed species, raw	3 oz.	82	1.7	15.7	0	0
Fish, seatrout, mixed species, raw	3 oz.	88	3.1	14.2	0	0
Fish, shad, raw	3 oz.	167	11.7	14.4	0	0
Fish, skipjack tuna, raw	3 oz.	88	0.9	18.7	0	0
Fish, snapper, mixed species, raw	3 oz.	85	1.1	17.4	0	0
Fish, striped bass, raw	3 oz.	82	2	15.1	0	0
Fish, striped mullet	3 oz.	99	3.2	16.4	0	0
Fish, sturgeon, mixed species, raw	3 oz.	89	3.4	13.7	0	0

F (cont.)

FOOD ITEM	Serving Size	Cal.	Fat	Protein	Carbs	Fiber
Fish, swordfish, raw	3 oz	103	3.4	16.8	0	0
Fish, trout, mixed species, raw	3 oz	126	5.6	17.7	0	0
Fish, white sucker, raw	3 oz	78	2	14.2	0	0
Fish, whitefish, raw	3 oz	114	5	16.2	0	0
Fish, wolffish, atlantic, raw	3 oz	82	2	14.9	0	0
Fish, yellowfin tuna, raw	3 oz	93	0.9	19.8	0	0
Fish, yellowtail, mixed species, raw	3 oz	124	4.5	19.7	0	0
Flan, caramel custard	5 1/2 oz.	303	12	4	43	0
Flaxseed	1 tbsp.	59	4.1	2.3	4.1	3.3
Flaxseed oil	1 tbsp.	120	13.6	0	0	0
Frankfurter	1 serving	151	13.4	5.3	2.2	0
Frankfurter, beef	1 frankfurter	188	16.9	6.4	2.3	0
Frankfurter, beef & pork	1 frankfurter	174	15.8	6.6	1	1.4
Frankfurter, chicken	1 frankfurter	116	8.8	5.8	3.1	0
Frankfurter, meat	1 frankfurter	151	13.4	5.3	2.2	0
Frankfurter, meatless	1 frankfurter	163	9.6	13.7	5.4	2.7
Frankfurter, pork	1 frankfurter	204	18	9.7	0.2	0.1
Frankfurter, turkey	1 frankfurter	102	8	6.4	0.7	0
French fries, frozen, unprepared, 18 fries	1 serving	170	6.7	2.8	27.7	3.4
French toast, frozen, ready-to-heat	1 piece	126	3.6	4.3	18.9	0.6
Frosting, creamy chocolate	2 tbsp	164	7.3	0.5	26.1	0.4
Frosting, creamy vanilla	2 tbsp	160	6.3	0	25.6	0
Frozen yogurt, chocolate, soft-serve	1/2 cup	115	4.3	2.9	17.9	1.6
Frozen yogurt, vanilla, soft-serve	1/2 cup	117	4	2.9	17.4	0
Fruit cocktail, canned	1 cup	229	0.2	1	59.5	2.9
Fruit punch, prepared from concentrate	8 fl oz.	124	0.5	0.2	30.2	0.2
Fruit salad, canned in syrup	1 cup	186	0.2	0.9	48.7	2.6
Fruit salad, canned in water	1 cup	74	0.2	0.9	19.3	2.5

G

FOOD ITEM	Serving Size	Cal.	Fat	Protein	Carbs	Fiber
Garden cress, raw	1 cup	16	0.3	1.3	2.7	0.6
Garlic	1 clove	4	0	0.2	1	0.1
Garlic powder	1 tsp	9	0	0.5	2	0.3
Gelatin dessert mix, prepared w/ water	1/2 cup	84	0	1.6	19.1	0

FOOD ITEM	Serving Size	Cal.	Fat	Protein	Carbs	Fiber
G (cont.)						
Gin, 80 Proof	1 fl oz.	73	0	0	0	0
Ginger root	1 tsp	2	0	0	0.4	0
Ginger, ground	1 tsp	6	0.1	0.2	1.3	0.2
Ginkgo nuts	1 oz	52	0.5	1.2	10.7	0
Ginkgo nuts, dried	1 oz	99	0.6	2.9	20.5	0
Goose liver, raw	1 liver	125	4	15.4	5.9	0
Goose, meat & skin, roasted	1 cup chopped	427	30.7	35.2	0	0
Goose, meat only, roasted	1 cup chopped	340	18.1	41.4	0	0
Gourd, white-flowered	1 gourd	108	0.2	4.8	26.1	0
Granola bars, hard, plain	1 bar	134	5.6	2.9	18.3	1.5
Granola bars, soft, plain	1 bar	126	4.9	2.1	19.1	1.3
Grape juice	8 fl oz.	160	0	0	40	0
Grapefruit	1/2 fruit	50	0	1	12	3
Grapefruit juice, sweetened	8 fl oz.	125	0	0	32.6	0
Grapefruit juice, unsweetened	8 fl oz.	91	0.2	1.2	21.5	0
Grapes, canned, heavy syrup	1 cup	187	0.3	1.2	50.3	1.5
Grapes, red or green	1 cup	106	0.2	1.1	27.9	1.4
Gravy, mushroom, canned	1 can	149	8.1	3.8	16.3	1.2
Gravy, au jus, canned	1 can	48	0.6	3.6	7.5	0
Gravy, beef, canned	1 can	154	6.9	10.9	14	1.2
Gravy, chicken, canned	1 can	235	17	5.8	16.2	1.2
Gravy, turkey, canned	1 can	152	6.2	7.7	15.2	1.2
Guacamole dip	2 tbsp	50	4	12	4	0
Guavas	1 fruit	37	0.5	1.4	7.8	3
H						
Ham, chopped	1 slice	50	2.9	4.6	1.2	0
Ham, minced	1 slice	55	4.3	3.4	0.4	0
Ham, sliced	1 slice	46	2.4	4.6	1.1	0.4
Hazlenuts, dry roasted	1 oz	183	17.7	4.2	5	2.7
Hazlenuts, blanched	1 oz	178	17.3	3.9	4.8	3.1
Hominy, canned, white	1 cup	119	1.5	2.4	23.5	4.1
Hominy, canned, yellow	1 cup	115	1.4	2.4	22.8	4
Honey	1 tbsp	64	0	0.1	17.3	0

FOOD ITEM	Serving Size	Cal.	Fat	Protein	Carbs	Fiber
H (cont.)						
Honeydew melons	1 cup, diced	61	0.2	0.9	15.5	1.4
Horseradish	1 tsp	2	0	0.1	0.6	0.2
Hot chocolate	8 fl oz.	200	10	9	25	3
Hummus	1 tbsp	23	1.3	1.1	2	0.8
Hush puppies	1 hush puppy	74	2.9	1.7	10.1	0.6
I						
Ice cream cone, rolled or sugar type	1 cone	40	0.4	0.8	8.4	0.2
Ice cream cone, wafer or cake type	1 cone	17	0.3	0.3	3.2	0.1
Ice cream, chocolate	1/2 cup	143	7.3	2.5	18.6	0.8
Ice cream, strawberry	1/2 cup	127	5.5	2.1	18.2	0.6
Ice cream, vanilla	1/2 cup	144	7.9	2.5	16.9	0.5
Iced tea, presweetened	8 fl oz.	100	0	0	25	0
Iced tea, unsweetened	8 fl oz.	2	0	0	0	0
Italian seasoning	1 tsp	4	0	0	1	0
J						
Jams and preserves	1 tbsp.	56	0	0.1	13.8	0.2
Japanese chestnuts	1 oz.	44	0.2	0.6	9.9	0
Japanese soba noodles, cooked	1 cup	113	0.1	5.7	24.4	1.7
Japanese ramen noodles, packaged, dry	1 serving	195	7.3	4	28	1
Jellies	1 tbsp.	55	0	0	14.4	0.2
K						
Kale	1 cup, chopped	34	0.5	2.2	6.7	1.3
Kiwifruit	1 medium	45	0	2	11	5
Kumquats	1 fruit	13	0.2	0.4	3	1.2
L						
Lamb, cubed, raw	1 oz.	38	1.5	5.7	0	0
Lamb, foreshank, raw	1 oz.	57	3.8	5.4	0	0
Lamb, ground, raw	1 oz.	80	6.6	4.7	0	0
Lamb, leg, shank half, raw	1 oz.	52	3.3	5.4	0	0
Lamb, leg, sirloin half, raw	1 oz.	74	5.9	4.9	0	0

FOOD ITEM

FOOD ITEM	Serving Size	Cal.	Fat	Protein	Carbs	Fiber
L (cont.)						
Lamb, leg, whole, choice, raw	1 oz.	65	4.8	5.1	0	0
Lamb, loin, choice, raw	1 oz.	79	6.4	4.9	0	0
Lamb, rib, choice, raw	1 oz.	97	8.7	4.3	0	0
Lamb, shoulder, arm, raw	1 oz.	69	5.4	4.9	0	0
Lamb, shoulder, blade, raw	1 oz.	69	5.4	4.8	0	0
Lamb, shoulder, whole, raw	1 oz.	69	5.4	4.8	0	0
Lard	1 tbsp.	115	12.8	0	0	0
Leeks	1 leek	54	0.3	1.3	12.6	1.6
Lemon juice	1 cup	61	0	0.9	21.1	1
Lemon juice, canned or bottled	1 tbsp.	3	0	0.1	1	0.1
Lemon pepper seasoning	1 tsp.	7	0	0	1	0
Lemonade powder	1 scoop	102	0	0	26.9	0
Lemonade, pink concentrate, prepared	8 fl oz.	99	0	0.2	25.9	0
Lemonade, white concentrate, prepared	8 fl oz.	131	0.1	0.2	34	0.2
Lemons w/ peel	1 fruit	22	0.3	1.3	11.6	5.1
Lentils, cooked	1 cup	230	0.7	17.8	39.8	15.6
Lentils, sprouted, raw	1 cup	82	0.4	6.9	17	0
Lettuce, green leaf	1 cup, shredded	5	0.1	0.5	1	0.5
Lettuce, iceberg	1 cup, shredded	10	0.1	0.7	2.2	0.9
Lettuce, red leaf	1 cup, shredded	3	0	0.2	0.4	0.2
Lettuce, romaine	1 cup, shredded	8	0.1	0.6	1.5	1
Lime juice	1 cup	62	0.2	1	20.7	1
Limes	1 fruit	20	0.1	0.5	7.1	1.9
Liverwurst, pork	1 slice	59	5.1	2.5	0.4	0
Lobster, northern, raw	1 lobster	135	1.3	28.2	0.8	0
Luncheon meat, beef, loaved	1 oz.	87	7.4	4.1	0.8	0
Luncheon meat, beef, thin sliced	1 oz.	50	1.1	8	1.6	0
Luncheon meat, meatless slices	1 slice	26	1.6	2.5	0.6	0
Luncheon meat, pork & chicken, minced	1 oz.	56	3.9	4.3	0.4	0
Luncheon meat, pork & ham, minced	1 oz.	88	7.45	3.75	1.3	0
Luncheon meat, pork or beef	1 oz.	99	9	3.5	0.6	0
Luncheon meat, pork, canned	1 oz.	95	8.6	3.5	0.6	0
Luncheon meat, pork, ham & chicken, minced	1 oz.	87	7.6	3.7	0.8	0
Luncheon sausage, pork & beef	1 oz.	74	5.9	4.3	0.4	0

FOOD ITEM	Serving Size	Cal.	Fat	Protein	Carbs	Fiber
M						
Macadamia nuts	1 oz. (10-12 nuts)	203	21.5	2.2	3.6	2.3
Macaroni and cheese, commercial, prepared	1 cup	259	2.6	11.3	47.5	1.5
Macaroni, cooked	1 cup	197	0.9	6.6	39.6	1.8
Malt drink mix, dry	3 heaping tsp	87	1.7	2.4	15.9	0.2
Malt beverage	8 fl oz.	144	0.2	0.7	32.2	0
Mangos	1 fruit	135	0.6	1.1	35.2	3.7
Maraschino cherries	1 cherry	8	0	0	2.1	0.2
Margarine, fat free spread	1 tbsp	6	0.4	0	0.6	0
Margarine, stick	1 tbsp	100	11.2	0	0.3	0
Margarine, stick, unsalted	1 tbsp	102	11.4	0.1	0.1	0
Margarine, tub	1 tbsp	102	11.4	0.1	0.1	0
Martini	1 fl oz.	69	0	0	0.6	0
Mayonnaise	1 tbsp	100	11	0	0	0
Milk, 1% low fat	1 cup	102	2.4	8.2	12.2	0
Milk, 2% low fat	1 cup	138	4.9	9.7	13.5	0
Milk, buttermilk, cultured, reduced fat	1 cup	137	4.9	10	13	0
Milk, chocolate	1 cup	208	8.5	7.9	25.9	2
Milk, dry, nonfat, instant	1/3 cup dry	82	0.1	8	12	0
Milk, evaporated	1/2 cup	169	9.5	8.5	12.6	0
Milk, skim or nonfat	1 cup	83	0.2	8.3	12.2	0
Milk, canned, sweetened condensed	1 cup	982	26.6	24.2	166.5	0
Milk, whole	1 cup	146	7.9	7.9	11	0
Milkshake, dry mix, vanilla	1 envelope packet	69	0.5	4.9	11.1	0.3
Millet	1 cup	756	8.4	22	145.7	17
Miso soup	1 cup	547	16.5	32.1	72.8	14.9
Mixed nuts	1 cup	814	70.5	23.7	34.7	12.3
Molasses	1 tablespoon	58	0	0	15	0
Muffins, apple bran	1 muffin	300	3	1	61	1
Muffins, banana nut	1 muffin	480	24	3	60	2
Muffins, blueberry	1 muffin	313	7.3	6.2	54.2	2.9
Muffins, chocolate chip	1 muffin	510	24	2	69	4
Muffins, corn	1 muffin	345	9.5	6.6	57.5	3.8
Muffins, oat bran	1 muffin	305	8.3	7.9	54.5	5.2
Muffins, plain	1 muffin	242	9.1	3.8	36.3	1.5

FOOD ITEM	Serving Size	Cal.	Fat	Protein	Carbs	Fiber
M (cont.)						
Mushrooms	1 cup, pieces	15	0.2	2.2	2.3	0.8
Mushrooms, enoki	1 large	2	0	0.1	0.4	0.1
Mushrooms, oyster	1 large	55	0.8	6.1	9.2	3.6
Mushrooms, portobello	1 large	0	0	0	0	0
Mushrooms, shiitake	1 mushroom	11	0	0.3	2.7	0.4
Mussels, blue, raw	1 cup	129	3.4	17.8	5.5	0
Mustard greens	1 cup, chopped	15	0.1	1.5	2.7	1.8
Mustard seed, yellow	1 tbsp	53	3.2	2.8	3.9	1.6
Mustard spinach	1 cup, chopped	33	0.5	3.3	5.9	4.2
Mustard, prepared, yellow	1 tsp	3	0.2	0.2	0.4	0.2
N						
Natto (fermented soybeans)	1 cup	371	19.3	31	25.1	9.5
Nectarines	1 fruit	60	0.4	1.4	14.3	2.3
New Zealand spinach	1 cup, chopped	8	0.1	0.8	1.4	0
Nutmeg, ground	1 tsp	12	0.8	0.1	1.1	0.5
O						
Oat bran	1 cup	231	6.6	16.3	62.2	14.5
Oatmeal, instant, prepared w/ water	1 cup	129	2.1	5.4	22.4	3.7
Oil, canola	1 tbsp	124	14	0	0	0
Oil, canola & soybean	1 tbsp	119	14	0	0	0
Oil, coconut	1 tbsp	120	13.6	0	0	0
Oil, corn, peanut & olive	1 tbsp	120	13.6	0	0	0
Oil, olive	1 tbsp	119	13.5	0	0	0
Oil, peanut	1 tbsp	119	13.5	0	0	0
Oil, sesame	1 tbsp	120	13.6	0	0	0
Oil, soy	1 tbsp	120	13.6	0	0	0
Oil, vegetable, almond	1 tbsp	120	13.6	0	0	0
Oil, vegetable, cocoa butter	1 tbsp	120	13.6	0	0	0
Oil, vegetable, coconut	1 tbsp	117	13.6	0	0	0
Oil, vegetable, grapeseed	1 tbsp	120	13.6	0	0	0
Oil, vegetable, hazelnut	1 tbsp	120	13.6	0	0	0
Oil, vegetable, nutmeg butter	1 tbsp	120	13.6	0	0	0

FOOD ITEM	Serving Size	Cal.	Fat	Protein	Carbs	Fiber
Oil, vegetable, palm	1 tbsp	120	13.6	0	0	0
Oil, vegetable, poppyseed	1 tbsp	120	13.6	0	0	0
Oil, vegetable, rice bran	1 tbsp	120	13.6	0	0	0
Oil, vegetable, sheanut	1 tbsp	120	13.6	0	0	0
Oil, vegetable, tomatoseed	1 tbsp	120	13.6	0	0	0
Oil, vegetable, walnut	1 tbsp	1927	218	0	0	0
Okra	1 cup	31	0.1	2	7	3.2
Onion powder	1 tsp	8	0	0.2	1.9	0.1
Onions	1 cup, chopped	67	0.1	1.5	16.2	2.2
Onions, sweet	1 onion	106	0.3	2.7	25	3
Orange juice	8 fl oz	109	0.6	1.9	25	0.5
Orange marmalade	1 tbsp	49	0	0.1	13.3	0.1
Oranges	1 large	86	0.2	1.7	21.6	4.4
Oregano, dried	1 tsp, ground	6	0.2	0.2	1.2	0.8
Oyster, eastern, raw	3 oz.	50	1.3	4.4	4.6	0
Oyster, pacific, raw	3 oz.	69	1.9	8	4.2	0

P

FOOD ITEM	Serving Size	Cal.	Fat	Protein	Carbs	Fiber
Pancakes, blueberry	1 pancake	84	3.5	2.3	11	0
Pancakes, buttermilk	1 pancake	86	3.5	2.6	10.9	0
Pancakes, plain, dry mix	1 pancake	74	1	2	13.9	0.5
Papayas	1 cup, cubed	55	0.2	0.9	13.7	2.5
Paprika	1 tsp	6	0.3	0.3	1.2	0.8
Parsley	1 cup	22	0.5	1.8	3.8	2
Parsley, dried	1 tsp	1	0	0.1	0.2	0.1
Parsnips	1 cup, sliced	100	0.4	1.6	23.9	6.5
Passion fruit	1 fruit	17	0.1	0.4	4.2	1.9
Pasta, corn, cooked	1 cup	176	1	3.6	39	6.7
Pasta, plain, cooked	1 cup	197	0.9	6.6	39.6	2.4
Pasta, spinach, cooked	1 cup	195	1.4	7.6	37.5	2.4
Pastrami, turkey	1 oz	40	1.8	5.2	0.5	0
Pate de foie gras	1 tbsp	60	5.7	1.5	0.6	0
Pate, chicken liver, canned	1 tbsp	26	1.7	1.7	0.9	0
Pate, goose liver, canned	1 tbsp	60	5.7	1.5	0.6	0
Peaches	1 large	61	0.4	1.4	15	2.4

FOOD ITEM

FOOD ITEM	Serving Size	Cal.	Fat	Protein	Carbs	Fiber
P (cont.)						
Peaches, canned	1 cup, halved	59	0.1	1.1	14.9	3.2
Peanut butter, chunky	2 tbsp	188	16	7.7	6.9	2.6
Peanut butter, smooth	2 tbsp	188	16.1	8	6.3	1.9
Peanuts, dry roasted w/ salt	1 oz	166	14	6.7	6.1	2.3
Peanuts, raw	1 oz	161	13.9	7.3	4.5	2.4
Pears	1 pear	121	0.3	0.8	32.3	6.5
Pears, asian	1 pear	116	0.6	1.4	29.3	9.9
Pears, canned	1 cup	71	0.1	0.5	19.1	3.9
Peas, green, fresh, cooked	1 cup	134	0.3	8.5	25	8.8
Peas, green, frozen, cooked	1 cup	125	0.4	8.2	22.8	8.8
Peas, split, cooked	1 cup	231	0.7	16.3	41.3	16.3
Pecans	1 oz. (20 halves)	196	20.4	2.6	3.9	2.7
Pepper, black	1 tsp	5	0.1	0.2	1.4	0.6
Pepper, red or cayenne	1 tsp	6	0.3	0.2	1	0.5
Pepperoni	15 slices	135	11.7	5.9	1.2	0.4
Peppers, chili, green	1 cup	29	0.4	1	6.4	2.4
Peppers, chili, red	1 pepper	18	0.2	0.8	4	0.7
Peppers, chili, sun-dried	1 pepper	2	0	0.1	0.4	0.2
Peppers, jalapeno	1 pepper	4	0.1	0.2	0.8	0.4
Peppers, sweet, green	1 medium	24	0.2	1	5.5	2
Peppers, sweet, red	1 medium	31	0.3	1.1	7.2	2.4
Peppers, sweet, yellow	1 medium	32	0.2	1.2	7.5	1.1
Persimmons	1 fruit	32	0.1	0.2	8.4	0
Pheasant, boneless, raw	1/2 pheasant	724	37.2	90.8	0	0
Pheasant, breast, skinless, boneless, raw	1/2 breast	242	5.9	44.4	0	0
Pheasant, leg, skinless, boneless, raw	1 leg	143	4.6	23.8	0	0
Pheasant, skinless, raw	1/2 pheasant	468	12.8	83	0	0
Pickle relish, sweet	1 tbsp	20	0.1	0.1	5.3	0.2
Pickle, sour	1 large 4"	15	0.3	0.4	3.1	1.6
Pickle, sweet	1 large 4"	158	0.3	0.5	42.9	1.5
Pickles, dill	1 large 4"	24	0.2	0.8	5.5	1.6
Pie crust, graham cracker, baked	1 pie crust	1037	52.3	8.8	136.9	3.2
Pie, apple	1 piece	411	19.4	3.7	57.5	0
Pie, blueberry	1 piece	290	12.5	2.2	43.6	1.3

FOOD ITEM	Serving Size	Cal.	Fat	Protein	Carbs	Fiber
P (cont.)						
Pie, cherry	1 piece	325	13.8	2.5	49.7	1
Pie, lemon meringue	1 piece	303	9.8	1.7	53.3	1.4
Pie, pecan	1 piece	452	20.9	4.5	64.6	4
Pie, pumpkin	1 piece	229	10.4	4.3	29.8	2.9
Pine nuts	1 oz. (167 kernels)	191	19.3	3.8	3.7	1
Pineapple	1 fruit	227	0.6	2.5	59.6	6.6
Pineapple, canned	1 slice	15	0	0.2	3.9	0.4
Pita bread, whole wheat	1 pita	170	1.7	6.4	35.2	4.8
Pistachio nuts	1 oz (49 kernels)	161	13	6	7.6	2.9
Pizza, cheese	1 slice (3.7 oz.)	250	10	11	29	2
Pizza, pepperoni	1 slice (3.7 oz.)	288	15.2	11.7	26.1	1.7
Plantains	1 medium	218	0.7	2.3	57.1	4.1
Plums	1 fruit	30	0.2	0.5	7.5	0.9
Plums, canned	1 plum	19	0	0.2	5.1	0.4
Polenta	1/2 cup	220	2	2	24	1
Pomegranates	1 fruit	105	0.5	1.5	26.4	0.9
Popcorn cakes	1 cake	38	0.3	1	8	0.3
Popcorn, air-popped	1 cup	31	0.3	1	6.2	1.2
Popcorn, caramel-coated	1 oz	122	3.6	1.1	22.4	1.5
Popcorn, cheese	1 cup	58	3.7	1	5.7	1.1
Popcorn, oil-popped	1 cup	55	3.1	1	6.3	1.1
Popovers, dry mix	1 oz	105	1.2	2.9	20	0.5
Poppy seed	1 tsp	15	1.3	0.5	0.7	0.3
Pork, cured, breakfast strips, cooked	3 slices	156	12.4	9.8	0.3	0
Pork, cured, ham, extra lean, canned	3 oz	116	4.1	17.9	0.4	0
Pork, cured, ham, patties	1 patty	205	18.4	8.3	1.1	0
Pork, cured, ham, extra lean, cooked	3 oz	140	6.5	18.6	0.4	0
Pork, cured, salt pork, raw	1 oz	212	22.8	1.4	0	0
Pork, fresh ground, cooked	3 oz	252	17.6	21.8	0	0
Pork, leg, rump half, cooked	3 oz	214	12.1	24.5	0	0
Pork, leg, shank half, cooked	3 oz	246	17	21.5	0	0
Pork, leg, whole, cooked	3 oz	232	14.9	22.8	0	0
Pork, loin, blade, cooked	3 oz	275	20.9	20.1	0	0
Pork, loin, center loin, cooked	3 oz	199	11.4	22.3	0	0

FOOD ITEM	Serving Size	Cal.	Fat	Protein	Carbs	Fiber
P (cont.)						
Pork, loin, center rib, cooked	3 oz	214	12.8	22.9	0	0
Pork, loin, sirloin, cooked	3 oz	176	8	24.2	0	0
Pork, loin, tenderloin, cooked	3 oz	147	5.1	23.6	0	0
Pork, loin, top loin, cooked	3 oz	192	9.7	24.4	0	0
Pork, loin, whole, cooked	3 oz	211	12.4	23	0	0
Pork, shoulder, arm, cooked	3 oz	238	18.1	17.3	0	0
Pork, shoulder, blade, cooked	3 oz	229	16	19.6	0	0
Pork, shoulder, whole, cooked	3 oz	248	18.2	19.8	0	0
Pork, spareribs, cooked	3 oz	337	25.7	24.7	0	0
Potato chips, barbecue	1 oz	139	9.2	2.2	14.9	1.2
Potato chips, cheese	1 oz	141	7.7	2.4	16.3	1.5
Potato chips, salted	1 oz	152	9.8	1.9	15	1.3
Potato chips, sour cream & onion	1 oz	151	9.6	2.3	14.6	1.5
Potato chips, reduced fat	1 oz	134	5.9	2	18.9	1.7
Potato chips, unsalted	1 oz	152	9.8	2	15	1.4
Potato flour	1 cup	571	0.5	11	132.9	9.4
Potato salad	1 cup	358	20.5	6.7	27.9	3.2
Potatoes	1 medium	164	0.2	4.3	37.2	4.7
Potatoes, baked, w/ skin	1 medium	160	0.2	4.3	36.5	3.8
Potatoes, baked, w/o skin	1 medium	143	0.2	2.8	33.3	3.3
Potatoes, mashed	1 cup	237	8.9	3.9	35.2	3.2
Potatoes, red	1 medium	153	0.3	4	33.9	3.6
Potatoes, russet	1 medium	168	0.2	4.6	38.5	2.8
Potatoes, scalloped	1 cup	211	9	7	26.4	4.7
Potatoes, white	1 medium	149	0.2	3.6	33.5	5.1
Pretzels, hard, plain, salted	1 oz	108	0.9	2.6	22.4	0.9
Prune juice	8 fl oz	180	0	2	43	3
Pudding, banana	1/2 cup	154	2.5	4	29	0
Pudding, chocolate	1/2 cup	154	2.8	4.6	27.7	0
Pudding, coconut cream	1/2 cup	157	3.3	4.2	28.2	0.1
Pudding, lemon	1/2 cup	157	2.5	4	29.7	0
Pudding, rice	1/2 cup	163	2.4	4.8	30.6	0.1
Pudding, tapioca	1/2 cup	154	2.4	4.2	28.7	0
Pudding, vanilla	1/2 cup	148	2.5	4.3	27.2	0

FOOD ITEM	Serving Size	Cal.	Fat	Protein	Carbs	Fiber
P (cont.)						
Pumpkin	1 cup	30	0.1	1.2	7.5	0.6
Pumpkin pie mix	1 cup	281	0.4	2.9	71.3	22.4
Pumpkin, canned	1 cup	83	0.7	2.7	19.8	7.1
R						
Rabbit, cooked	3 oz	167	6.8	24.7	0	0
Radicchio	1 cup, shredded	9	0.1	0.6	1.8	0.4
Radishes	1 cup, sliced	19	0.1	0.8	3.9	1.9
Raisins	1 1/2 oz	129	0.2	1.3	34	1.6
Raisins, golden	1 1/2 oz	130	0.2	1.4	34.1	1.7
Raspberries	1 cup	64	0.8	1.5	14.7	8
Rhubarb	1 cup, diced	26	0.2	1.1	5.5	2.2
Rice cakes, brown rice, corn	1 cake	35	0.3	0.8	7.3	0.3
Rice cakes, brown rice, multigrain	1 cake	35	0.3	0.8	7.2	0.3
Rice cakes, brown rice, plain	1 cake	35	0.3	0.7	7.3	0.4
Rice, brown, cooked	1 cup	218	1.6	4.5	45.8	3.5
Rice, white, cooked	1 cup	242	0.3	4.4	53.2	0.6
Rice, wild	1 cup	166	0.5	6.5	35	3
Rolls, dinner	1 roll	136	3.1	3.6	22.9	0.8
Rolls, dinner, wheat	1 roll	117	2.7	3.7	19.7	1.6
Rolls, dinner, whole-wheat	1 roll	114	2	3.7	21.9	3.2
Rolls, french	1 roll	119	1.8	3.7	21.5	0.1
Rolls, hamburger or hotdog	1 roll	120	1.9	4.1	21.3	0.9
Rolls, hard (incl. kaiser)	1 roll	126	1.8	4.2	22.6	1
Rolls, pumpernickel	1 roll	119	1.2	4.6	22.7	2.3
Rosemary	1 tsp	1	0	0	0.1	0.1
Rosemary, dried	1 tsp	4	0.2	0.1	0.8	0.5
Rum, 80 proof	1 fl oz.	64	0	0	0	0
Rutabagas	1 cup, cubed	50	0.3	1.7	11.4	3.5
Rye	1 cup	566	4.2	24.9	117.9	24.7
Rye flour, dark	1 cup	415	3.4	18	88	28.9
Rye flour, light	1 cup	374	1.4	8.6	81.8	14.9
Rye flour, medium	1 cup	361	1.8	9.6	79	14.9

FOOD ITEM	Serving Size	Cal.	Fat	Protein	Carbs	Fiber
S						
Sage, ground	1 tsp.	2	0.1	0.1	0.4	0.3
Sake	1 fl oz.	39	0	0.1	1.5	0
Salad dressing, 1000 island	1 tbsp.	58	5.5	0.2	2.3	0.1
Salad dressing, bacon & tomato	1 tbsp.	49	5.3	0.3	0.3	0
Salad dressing, blue cheese	1 tbsp.	77	8	0.7	1.1	0
Salad dressing, caesar	1 tbsp.	78	8.5	0.2	0.5	0
Salad dressing, coleslaw	1 tbsp.	61	5.2	0.1	3.7	0
Salad dressing, french	1 tbsp.	71	7	0.1	2.4	0
Salad dressing, honey dijon	1 tbsp.	57.5	5	0.5	3	0.5
Salad dressing, italian	1 tbsp.	43	4.2	0.1	1.5	0
Salad dressing, mayo-based	1 tbsp.	57	4.9	0.1	3.5	0
Salad dressing, mayonnaise	1 tbsp.	103	11.7	0	0	0
Salad dressing, peppercorn	1 tbsp.	76	8.2	0.2	0.5	0
Salad dressing, ranch	1 tbsp.	25	0	0	0	0
Salad dressing, russian	1 tbsp.	76	7.8	0.2	1.6	0
Salad, chicken	6 oz.	420	33	45	11	1.5
Salad, egg	6 oz.	300	23	20	14	0.5
Salad, prima pasta	6 oz.	360	30	4.8	18	2.5
Salad, seafood w/ crab & shrimp	6 oz.	420	34	0	20	0
Salad, tuna	6 oz.	450	36	16	14	0
Salami, cooked, turkey	1 oz.	37.7	2.3	0.7	0	0
Salami, dry, pork or beef	3 slices	104	8.1	6.3	1	0
Salami, italian pork	1 oz.	119	10.4	6.1	0.3	0
Salsa, w/ oil	2 tbsp.	40	3	0	8	0
Salsa, w/o oil	2 tbsp.	15	0	0	3.5	0
Salt	1 tbsp.	0	0	0	0	0
Sauce, alfredo	1/4 cup	120	11	15	3	2
Sauce, barbecue	1 cup	188	4.5	4.5	32	3
Sauce, cheese	1 cup	479	36.3	25.1	13.3	0.2
Sauce, cranberry	1 cup	418	0.4	0.6	107.8	2.8
Sauce, hollandaise	1 cup	62	1.5	2.3	10.3	0.2
Sauce, honey mustard	1 tbsp.	30	1	0	5	0
Sauce, marinara	1 cup	185	6	4.9	28.2	1
Sauce, salsa	1 cup	70	0.4	4	16.2	4.1

FOOD ITEM	Serving Size	Cal.	Fat	Protein	Carbs	Fiber
S (cont.)						
Sauce, soy	1 tbsp.	10	0	0	0	0
Sauce, steak	1 tbsp.	25	0	0	6	0
Sauce, teriyaki	1 tbsp.	15	0	17	2	0
Sauce, tomato chili	1 cup	284	0.8	6.8	54	16.1
Sauce, worcestershire	1 cup	184	0	0	53.5	0
Sauerkraut	1/2 cup	25	0	1	5	4
Sausage, italian pork, raw	1 link	391	35.4	16.1	0.7	0
Sausage, pork	1 link	85	7.4	4.2	0	0
Sausage, smoked linked, pork	1 link	265	21.6	15.1	1.4	0
Sausage, turkey	1 link	0	0	0	0	0
Savory, ground	1 tsp.	4	0.1	0.1	1	0.6
Scallops	1 scallop	26	0.2	5	0.7	0
Seaweed, dried	1 oz.	50	0	0	13	0
Sesame seeds, dried	1 tbsp.	52	4.5	1.6	2.1	1.1
Shallots	1 tbsp, chopped	7	0	0.3	1.7	0
Shortening	1 tbsp.	113	12.8	0	0	0
Shrimp, mixed species, raw	1 medium piece	6	0.1	1.2	0.1	0
Snacks, cheese puffs or twists	1 oz.	157	9.7	2.1	15.2	0.3
Soda, club	12 fl oz.	0	0	0	0	0
Soda, cream	12 fl oz.	252	0	0	65.7	0
Soda, diet cola	12 fl oz.	0	0	0	0	0
Soda, ginger ale	12 fl oz.	166	0	0	42.8	0
Soda, lemon-lime	12 fl oz.	196	0	0	51.1	0
Soda, regular, w/ caffeine	12 fl oz.	155	0	0.2	39.8	0
Soda, regular, w/o caffeine	12 fl oz.	207	0	0.2	52.9	0
Soda, root beer	12 fl oz.	202	0	0	52.3	0
Soda, tonic water	12 fl oz.	166	0	0	42.9	0
Soup, beef broth	1 cup	29	0	5.3	1.7	0
Soup, beef stroganoff	1 cup	235	11	12.2	21.6	1.4
Soup, beef vegetable	1 cup	82	1.9	2.9	13.1	0.5
Soup, chicken broth	1 cup	39	1.3	4.9	0.9	0
Soup, chicken noodle	1 cup	75	2.4	4	9.3	0.7
Soup, chicken vegetable	1 cup	75	2.8	3.6	8.5	1
Soup, chicken w/ dumplings	1 cup	96	5.5	5.6	6	0.5

FOOD ITEM	Serving Size	Cal.	Fat	Protein	Carbs	Fiber
S (cont.)						
Soup, clam chowder	1 cup	95	2.8	4.8	12.4	1.5
Soup, cream of chicken	1 cup	117	7.3	3.4	9.2	0.2
Soup, cream of mushroom	1 cup	129	8.9	2.3	9.3	0.5
Soup, cream of potato	1 cup	149	6.4	5.7	17	0.5
Soup, minestrone	1 cup	82	2.5	4.2	11.2	1
Soup, split-pea w/ham	1 cup	190	4.4	10.3	27.9	2.3
Soup, tomato	1 cup	161	6	6.1	22.3	2.7
Soup, vegetarian	1 cup	72	1.9	2.1	11.9	0.5
Sour cream	1 tbsp	26	2.5	0.4	0.5	0
Sour cream, fat free	1 tbsp	9	0	0.3	1.8	0
Sour cream, reduced fat	1 tbsp	22	1.7	0.8	0.8	0
Soy milk	1 cup	127	4.7	10.9	12	3.2
Soy protein isolate	1 oz	96	1	22.9	2.1	1.6
Soybeans, green, cooked	1 cup	254	11.5	22.2	19.8	7.6
Soybeans, nuts, roasted	1/4 cup	194	9.2	17	14	3.4
Soyburger	1 patty	125	4.1	12.5	9.3	3.2
Spaghetti, cooked	1 cup	197	0.9	6.6	39.6	2.4
Spaghetti, spinach, cooked	1 cup	182	0.8	6.4	36.6	2.4
Spaghetti, whole-wheat, cooked	1 cup	174	0.7	7.4	37.1	6.3
Spinach	1 cup	7	0.1	0.9	1.1	0.7
Squab, boneless, raw	1 squab	585	47.4	36.8	0	0
Squab, skinless, raw	1 squab	239	12.6	29.4	0	0
Squash, summer	1 cup, sliced	18	0.2	1.4	3.8	1.2
Squash, winter	1 cup, cubed	39	0.2	1.1	10	1.7
Squid, mixed species, raw	1 oz	26	0.4	4.4	0.9	0
Stock, beef	1 cup	31	0.2	4.7	2.9	0
Stock, chicken	1 cup	86	2.9	6	8.5	0
Stock, fish	1 cup	40	1.9	5.3	0	0
Strawberries	1 cup	49	0.5	1	11.7	3
Succotash	1 piece	0	0	0	0	0
Sugar, brown	1 tsp	12	0	0	3.1	0
Sugar, granulated	1 tsp	16	0	0	4.2	0
Sugar, maple	1 tsp	11	0	0	2.7	0
Sugar, powdered	1 tsp	10	0	0	2.5	0

FOOD ITEM	Serving Size	Cal.	Fat	Protein	Carbs	Fiber
S (cont.)						
Sunflower seeds	1 tbsp	45	10	4	1.5	5
Sweet potato	1 cup, cubed	114	0.1	2.1	26.8	4
Syrup, chocolate	1 tbsp	66.5	1.7	0.8	11.9	0.5
Syrup, dark corn	1 tbsp	57	0	0	15.5	0
Syrup, grenadine	1 tbsp	53	0	0	13.3	0
Syrup, light corn	1 tbsp	59	0	0	15.9	0
Syrup, maple	1 tbsp	52	0	0	13.4	0
Syrup, pancake	1 tbsp	47	0	0	12.3	0.1
T						
Taco shell, hard	1 shell	55	3	2	6	0
Tangerines	1 large	52	0.3	0.8	13.1	1.8
Tarragon, dried	1 tsp	2	0	0.1	0.3	0
Tea, instant	1 cup	2	0	0.1	0.4	0
Thyme	1 tsp	1	0	0	0.2	0.1
Thyme, dried	1 tsp	3	0.1	0.1	0.6	0.4
Tofu, firm	1/2 cup	183	11	19.9	5.4	2.9
Tofu, fried	1 piece	35	2.6	2.2	1.4	0.5
Tofu, soft	1/2 cup	75.5	4.6	8.1	2.2	0.2
Tomato juice, canned, with salt	6 fl oz	31	0.1	1.4	7.7	0.7
Tomato juice, canned, without salt	6 fl oz	30	0.1	1.2	7.8	0.7
Tomato paste, canned	1/2 cup	107	0.6	5.7	24.8	5.9
Tomato sauce, canned	1 cup	78	0.6	3.2	18.1	3.7
Tomatoes, canned, crushed	1 cup	82	0.7	4.2	18.6	4.8
Tomatoes, green	1 cup, chopped	41	0.4	2.2	9.2	2
Tomatoes, orange	1 cup, chopped	25	0.3	1.8	5	1.4
Tomatoes, red	1 cup, chopped	32	0.4	1.6	7.1	2.2
Tomatoes, sun-dried	1 cup, chopped	139	1.6	7.6	30.1	6.6
Toppings, butterscotch or caramel	2 tbsp	103	0	0.6	27	0.4
Toppings, marshmallow cream	2 tbsp	132	0.1	0.3	32.3	0
Toppings, nuts in syrup	2 tbsp	184	9	1.8	23.8	0.9
Toppings, pineapple	2 tbsp	106	0	0	27.9	0.2
Toppings, strawberry	2 tbsp	107	0	0.1	27.8	0.3
Tortilla chips, plain	1 oz	142	7.4	1.9	17.8	1.8

FOOD ITEM	Serving Size	Cal.	Fat	Protein	Carbs	Fiber
Tortilla, corn	1 tortilla	45	0.5	2	9	3
Tortilla, flour	1 tortilla	160	3	18	28	3
Trail mix	1/4 cup	173.2	11	5	16.8	3
Turkey, deli sliced, white meat	1 oz.	30	1	5	0.5	0
Turkey, back, skinless, boneless, raw	1/2 back	180	5.3	31	0	0
Turkey, breast, boneless, raw	1/2 breast	541	11.5	102.9	0	0
Turkey, breast, skinless, boneless, raw	1/2 breast	433	2.5	95.9	0	0
Turkey, dark meat, boneless, raw	1/2 turkey	686	25.5	106.7	0	0
Turkey, dark meat, skinless, boneless, raw	1/2 turkey	532	12.8	98	0	0
Turkey, leg, boneless, raw	1 leg	412	12.5	70.3	0	0
Turkey, leg, skinless, boneless, raw	1 leg	355	7.8	67	0	0
Turkey, wing, boneless, raw	1 wing	204	9.9	26.7	0	0
Turkey, wing, skinless, boneless, raw	1 wing	95	1	20.2	0	0
Turkey, young hen, back, boneless, raw	1/2 back	650	47.5	52.2	0	0
Turkey, young hen, breast, boneless, raw	1/2 breast	1460	72.5	189	0	0
Turkey, young hen, dark meat, boneless, raw	1/2 turkey	1056	39.6	163	0	0
Turkey, young hen, leg, boneless, raw	1 leg	991	49.2	127.7	0	0
Turkey, young hen, wing, boneless, raw	1 wing	470	31.1	44.6	0	0
Turkey, young tom, back, boneless, raw	1/2 back	938	58.4	96.8	0	0
Turkey, young tom, breast, boneless, raw	1/2 breast	2701	113.4	392.9	0	0
Turkey, young tom, dark meat, boneless, raw	1/2 turkey	1884	63	307	0	0
Turkey, young tom, leg, boneless, raw	1 leg	1740	78.2	241.1	0	0
Turkey, young tom, wing, boneless, raw	1 wing	654	39	71.2	0	0
Turnip greens	1 cup, chopped	18	0.2	0.8	3.9	1.8
Turnips	1 cup, cubed	36	0.1	1.2	8.4	2.3

V

FOOD ITEM	Serving Size	Cal.	Fat	Protein	Carbs	Fiber
Vanilla extract	1 tbsp.	37	0	0	1.6	0
Veal, breast, raw	1 oz	59	4.2	5	0	0
Veal, cubed, raw	1 oz	31	0.7	5.7	0	0
Veal, ground, raw	1 oz	41	1.9	5.5	0	0
Veal, leg, raw	1 oz	33	0.9	5.9	0	0
Veal, loin, raw	1 oz	46	2.6	5.4	0	0
Veal, rib, raw	1 oz	46	2.6	5.3	0	0
Veal, shank, raw	1 oz	32	1	5.4	0	0

FOOD ITEM	Serving Size	Cal.	Fat	Protein	Carbs	Fiber
Veal, shoulder, arm, raw	1 oz	37	1.5	5.5	0	0
Veal, shoulder, blade, raw	1 oz	37	1.5	5.5	0	0
Veal, shoulder, whole, raw	1 oz	37	1.5	5.5	0	0
Veal, sirloin, raw	1 oz	43	2.2	5.4	0	0
Vegetable juice	8 fl oz	50	0	2	12	2
Vinegar	1 tbsp	2	0	0	0.8	0

W

FOOD ITEM	Serving Size	Cal.	Fat	Protein	Carbs	Fiber
Waffles, plain	1 waffle	218	10.6	5.9	24.7	0
Walnuts	1 oz. (14 halves)	185	18.5	4.3	3.9	1.9
Wasabi root	1 cup, sliced	142	0.8	6.2	30.6	10.1
Water chestnuts, chinese	1/2 cup, sliced	60	0.1	0.9	14.8	1.9
Watercress	1 cup, chopped	4	0	0.8	0.4	0.2
Watermelon	1 cup, diced	46	0.2	0.9	11.5	0.6
Wheat bran	1 cup	125	2.5	9	37.4	24.8
Wheat flour, whole grain	1 cup	407	2.2	16.4	87.1	14.6
Wheat germ	1 cup	414	11.2	26.6	59.6	15.2
Whipped cream	1 cup	154	13.3	1.9	7.5	0
Wine, cooking	1 tsp	2	0	0	0.3	0
Wine, red	3-1/2 oz. glass	74	0	0.2	1.8	0
Wine, rose	3-1/2 oz. glass	73	0	0.2	1.4	0
Wine, white	3-1/2 oz. glass	70	0	0.1	0.8	0
Yam	1 cup, cubed	177	0.3	2.3	41.8	6.1
Yeast, active, dry	1 tsp	12	0.2	1.5	1.5	0.8
Yogurt, fruit, low fat	8 oz. container	118	0.3	5.5	23.8	0
Yogurt, fruit, whole milk	8 oz. container	250	6	9	38	0
Yogurt, plain, low fat	8 oz. container	110	4	7.9	7	0
Yogurt, plain, whole milk	8 oz. container	138	7.4	12	10.6	0

Z

FOOD ITEM	Serving Size	Cal.	Fat	Protein	Carbs	Fiber
Zucchini	1 medium	45	0	2	10	1

Great Titles in the
SIMPLE PRINCIPLES™ SERIES

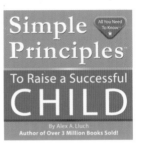

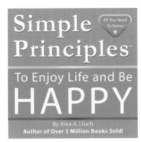

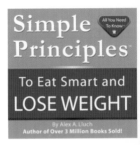

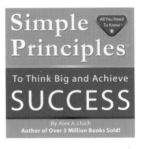

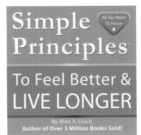

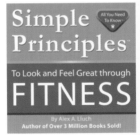

More Great Titles in the
SIMPLE PRINCIPLES™ SERIES

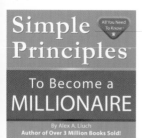

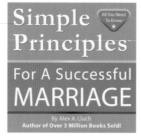

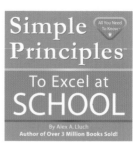

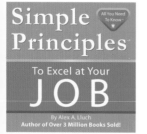

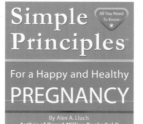

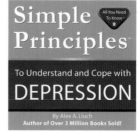

LOG ON TO **WSPUBLISHINGGROUP.COM** TO CHECK FOR RELEASE DATES ON THESE AND FUTURE TITLES.

Other Best-Selling Books
by Alex A. Lluch

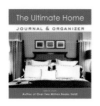

HOME & FINANCE
- The Very Best Home Improvement Guide & Document Organizer
- The Very Best Home Buying Guide & Document Organizer
- The Very Best Home Selling Guide & Document Organizer
- The Very Best Budget & Finance Guide with Document Organizer
- The Ultimate Home Journal & Organizer
- The Ultimate Home Buying Guide & Organizer

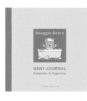

BABY JOURNALS & PARENTING
- The Complete Baby Journal Organizer & Keepsake
- Keepsake of Love Baby Journal
- Snuggle Bears Baby Journal Keepsake & Organizer
- Humble Bumbles Baby Journal
- Simple Principles to Raise a Successful Child

CHILDREN'S BOOKS
- I Like to Learn: Alphabet, Numbers, Colors & Opposites
- Alexander, It's Time for Bed!
- Do I Look Good in Color?
- Zoo Clues Animal Alphabet
- Animal Alphabet: Slide & Seek the ABC's
- Counting Chameleon
- Big Bugs, Small Bugs

Log on to **WSPublishingGroup.com** to check for release dates on these and future titles.

More Best-Selling Books by Alex A. Lluch

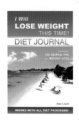

COOKING, FITNESS & DIET

- The Very Best Cooking Guide & Recipe Organizer
- Easy Cooking Guide & Recipe Organizer
- Get Fit Now! Workout Journal
- Lose Weight Now! Diet Journal & Organizer
- I Will Lose Weight This Time! Diet Journal
- The Ultimate Pocket Diet Journal

WEDDING PLANNING

- The Ultimate Wedding Planning Kit
- The Complete Wedding Planner & Organizer
- Easy Wedding Planner, Organizer & Keepsake
- Easy Wedding Planning Plus
- Easy Wedding Planning
- The Ultimate Wedding Workbook & Organizer
- The Ultimate Wedding Planner & Organizer
- Making Your Wedding Beautiful, Memorable & Unique
- Planning the Most Memorable Wedding on Any Budget
- My Wedding Journal, Organizer & Keepsake
- The Ultimate Wedding Planning Guide
- The Ultimate Guide to Wedding Music
- Wedding Party Responsibility Cards

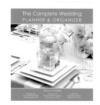

LOG ON TO **WSPublishingGroup.com** TO CHECK FOR RELEASE DATES ON THESE AND FUTURE TITLES.

About the Author and Creator of the
SIMPLE PRINCIPLES™ SERIES

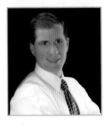

Alex A. Lluch is a seasoned entrepreneur with outstanding life achievements. He grew up very poor and lost his father at age 15. But through hard work and dedication, he has become one of the most successful authors and businessmen of our time. He is now using his life experience to write the simple principles™ series to help people improve their lives.

The following are a few of Alex's achievements:

- Author of over 3 million books sold in a wide range of categories: health, fitness, diet, home, finance, weddings, children, and babies
- President of WS Publishing Group, a successful publishing company
- President of WeddingSolutions.com, one of the world's most popular wedding planning websites
- President of UltimateGiftRegistry.com, an extensive website that allows users to register for gifts for all occasions
- President of a highly successful toy and candy company
- Has worked extensively in China, Hong Kong, Spain, Israel and Mexico
- Designed complex communication systems for Fortune 500 companies
- Black belt in Karate and Judo, winning many national tournaments
- Owns real estate in California, Colorado, Georgia and Montana
- B.S. in Electronics Engineering and an M.S. in Computer Science

Alex Lluch lives in San Diego, California with his wife of 16 years and their three wonderful children.

About the Co-Author

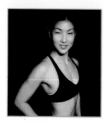

Sarah Jang is a true expert in eating smart and losing weight. During her childhood, she struggled with obesity. Like many Americans, Sarah tried every diet, but the more she tried to lose weight the more she would gain. She lived in a constant state of suffering, guilt, and shame. Her failure to lose weight led Sarah down a horrific, self-destructive path.

Her determination to "suffer no more" led Sarah to read countless books on weight loss and to work with many experts in the field.

During her research, she compiled a list of simple principles for eating smart and losing weight. These principles allowed Sarah to lose all her unwanted weight quickly and easily. Practicing these simple principles™ has allowed Sarah to stay slim, healthy, and fit for many years.

Now in her 30s, Sarah is in the best shape of her life. She is now sharing her expertise and years of research in eating smart and losing weight with the simple principles™ contained in this book.

Sarah graduated summa cum laude from Loyola University in Chicago with a bachelor's degree in Fine Arts. She now coaches others in weight loss and fitness.

Sarah Jang lives in San Diego, California where she enjoys a successful business career.